Self-Assessment in Haematology

Chris Pallister

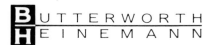

Butterworth-Heinemann Ltd
Linacre House, Jordan Hill, Oxford OX2 8DP

 PART OF REED INTERNATIONAL BOOKS

OXFORD   LONDON   BOSTON
MUNICH   NEW DELHI   SINGAPORE   SYDNEY
TOKYO   TORONTO   WELLINGTON

First published 1991

British Library Cataloguing in Publication Data
Pallister, Chris
  Self-assessment in haematology.
  I. Title
  616.1

ISBN 0 7506 1216 9

Library of Congress Cataloguing in Publication Data
Pallister, Chris
  Self-assessment in haematology / Chris Pallister.
    p.   cm.
  Includes bibliographical references.
  ISBN 0 7506 1216 9
  1. Hematology—Examinations, questions, etc.   I. Title.
  [DNLM: 1. Hematology—case studies.   2 Hematology—examination
  questions.   WH 18 P168s]
  RB145.P25   1991
  616.1'5'0076—dc20
  DNLM/DLC   91-26592
  for Library of Congress   CIP

Printed and bound in Great Britain by
Redwood Press Limited, Melksham, Wiltshire

Contents

Foreword

Multiple choice questions of one style or another are an established component of many modern examination schemes. In addition, the interpretation of laboratory and clinical data, in what have commonly been called "case studies", is becoming an increasingly popular means of assessing competence in medical laboratory sciences. Carefully constructed questions of this nature not only test straightforward recall of factual knowledge but also examine the wider understanding of a particular topic and the ability to assimilate laboratory and clinical information. These skills are now widely appreciated as important in a contemporary laboratory where major scientific advances are continually leading to significant improvements in diagnostic and therapeutic capabilities.

This present compendium offers an extensive range of questions in the diverse, general and specialised aspects of laboratory haematology. The questions have been compiled by an experienced teacher and practitioner of medical laboratory haematology. They are written in a consistent format, common to the majority of current examinations of this type, and are constructed primarily to assist students with their revision rather than to give typical examples of what might be expected in a formal examination paper. It should especially be emphasised, therefore, that students must not be tempted to memorise any of the questions. Specific examination questions from different examining bodies will vary both in content and in wording, and the precise wording of an individual question is, of course, crucial. Readers are encouraged to attempt the questions without guessing. Guessing in actual laboratory practice is dangerous at the very least, and most examiners penalise incorrect answers by some form of negative marking.

Answers, together with pertinent comments pointing to possible pitfalls, are provided at the end of each set of questions. Most benefit will be derived, however, by those who try to answer the questions without cheating. It is conceivable, and perhaps should be expected, that readers will not know or will disagree with some of the suggested answers. In those circumstances reference to reliable text books is recommended, in order to expand the correct response or to reconcile the differences. Used in this way, the broad collection of questions contained in this relatively concise volume will provide an extremely useful adjunct to a detailed revision schedule. In most instances the author cites the source of his own information and suggests further reading.

The overall aim of the book should be seen to inspire confidence rather than to frighten the reader. There are no devious or "trick" questions, and careful reasoning will usually prompt a logical response. The author implies that the book is directed towards those undertaking HNC/D, BSc and FIMLS courses. It is most likely, however, that students in all areas of laboratory haematology, clinical, diagnostic and research, will find the text both challenging and rewarding.

J.C. Giddings,
Haematology Department,
University of Wales College of Medicine,
Heath Park,
Cardiff,
UK.

Preface

γνῶθι σεαντον.

Know thyself.

Inscribed on the temple of Apollo
at Delphi.

In undertaking any course of study, it is prudent to continually monitor
one's progress. This is especially true of part time courses where access
to tutorial advice may be limited. Most students experience self-doubt
and even anxiety as examinations approach, but judicious application of
self-assessment techniques throughout the study period can help to
prevent, or at least alleviate, these feelings. It will provide evidence of
improvement in knowledge and skills as the course progresses and act as
a spur to further study. Equally importantly, it will help to prevent
complacency by highlighting gaps in one's knowledge. It can thus be
used as a guide to required study.

This book is designed to be used as part of such a process of
self-assessment for students of haematology. It should prove useful to
students of HNC/D, BSc, Fellowship of the IMLS and MSc courses. It
should also be of value for medical staff studying for membership of the
Royal College of Pathologists. Finally, I hope that it will prove an
interesting challenge to practising haematologists who worry that their
knowledge may be becoming rusty!

The book is divided into two parts: the first partconsists of a series
of graded multiple choice tests and the second is based on case studies.
Answers and short explanatory notes are included, where appropriate.
No attempt is made to provide more than the barest of reminders about
the answers. Suggestions for further reading are included as a guide to
further study, if required.

I am indebted to Mrs. G. Lee and Dr. R. Slade of the Department of
Haematology, Southmead Hospital, Bristol and Mrs. D. Reeves, Bristol
Polytechnic HEC for their skill, care and patience in checking the drafts

of this book. Without their help and advice, this book would have been much poorer. I am also, as ever, grateful to my wife for her patience and unfailing support during the book's preparation.

Bristol, 1991

C.J.P.

Part One
Multiple Choice Tests

Introduction

Completion and Scoring of the Multiple Choice Tests

The time allowed for the completion of each test is 60 minutes. Set aside sufficient time in a quiet room where you will not be disturbed for the duration of the test.

Each question consists of one stem and five items (marked A, B, C etc). Mark each item True, False, or Don't Know. The items in each question may be all true, all false, or any combination of true and false.

Complete each test before checking the answers. A correct answer scores 1 mark; an incorrect answer scores -1 mark and a don't know scores 0 marks.

Example

Q1.1   The following cars are manufactured by Austin Rover.
   A. Escort.
   B. Golf.
   C. Maestro.
   D. Sierra.
   E. Montego.

Your Answers	Correct Answers	Score
A. True.	False.	-1
B. False.	False.	1
C. Don't Know.	True.	0
D. True.	False.	-1
E. True.	True.	1
	Total Score	0

All of the questions in this book have been validated by HNC/D, BSc and FIMLS students to assess their level of difficulty and lack of ambiguity. As an approximate guide, a good final year HNC/D student should consistently score about 40% in a series of tests while an FIMLS or MSc student should expect to score consistently above 80%.

Hints on Successful Completion of the Multiple Choice Tests

If these tests are to be used for the purpose of self-assessment, care must be taken to avoid losing marks unnecessarily. Read each question carefully and make quite sure that it is clear what is being asked before attempting to answer. There are no "trick" questions in this book. Great care has been taken to avoid ambiguity and to exclude hidden meanings. For many of the questions, it is important that the precise meaning of words in the stem is understood. For example, a *characteristic* finding in a given disease is one which, if it were absent, would call the diagnosis into question. On the other hand, a *recognised* finding is one which is associated with the given condition but is not necessarily characteristic.

Each item in a question is independent of the others. There is no pattern to the number of true and false responses in a test, so don't waste time (and marks) looking for one.

Do **not** guess or mark randomly, but don't give up too easily either. Some of the questions are designed to require careful thought; the answer may become apparent if time is taken to think about it.

Suggested Reading

The answers provided to the multiple choice tests are deliberately brief. If this explanation is inadequate, a reference for further reading is provided in each case. It is suggested that these references be used in one of two ways; either as a source of further explanation of an answer or as a guide to further in-depth study of the subject. In the latter case, the suggested reference should be read carefully and then used to provide further sources of information. The suggested reading list is deliberately short. Each book was chosen for its suitability both as a fairly comprehensive text and as a primary resource.

If further study is undertaken, it may be instructive to repeat the tests to assess the efficacy of that study. However, it must be emphasised that a book such as this can only act as a *guide* to current levels of knowledge and must be interpreted with caution. No guarantee of pass marks can be given!

Eastham, R.D., *1991, Clinical Haematology* (7th ed.), Wright, Bristol.

Chanarin, I., 1990, *Laboratory Haematology*, Churchill Livingstone, Edinburgh.

Hall, R. and Malia R.G., 1991, *Medical Laboratory Haematology* (2nd ed.), Butterworths, London.

Hoffbrand, A.V. (ed.), 1985,*Recent Advances in Haematology 4*, Churchill Livingstone, Edinburgh.

Hoffbrand, A.V. (ed.), 1988,*Recent Advances in Haematology 5*, Churchill Livingstone, Edinburgh.

Hoffbrand, A.V. and Lewis, S.M. (eds), 1991, *Postgraduate Haematology* (3rd ed.), Heinemann, Oxford.

Roitt, I., Brostoff, J. and Male, D., 1990, *Immunology*, (2nd ed.), Churchill Livingstone, Edinburgh.

Multiple Choice Test One

Q1.1 **Severe deficiency of the following coagulation factors causes prolongation of the prothrombin time:**

A. factor I (fibrinogen).
B. factor XII.
C. factor V.
D. factor VII.
E. factor XIII.

Q1.2 **The following statements relate to the distribution of body iron in a healthy 70 kg adult male:**

A. circulating haemoglobin accounts for about 10% of the total body iron.
B. body stores account for at least 50% of the total.
C. muscle myoglobin accounts for up to 10% of the total.
D. plasma iron accounts for less than 0.1% of the total.
E. total body iron amounts to 30-40 mg.

Q1.3 **The following statements relate to vitamin B_{12}:**

A. poor diet is the commonest cause of deficiency in the UK.
B. total body stores in a 70 kg adult amount to about 3 mg.
C. it is absorbed maximally from the duodenum.
D. vegetables are a rich dietary source of vitamin B_{12}.
E. deficiency typically results in microcytic anaemia.

Q1.4 **The following substances are haem precursors:**

A. alanine.
B. δ-aminolaevulinic acid.
C. stercobilin.
D. glycine.
E. bilirubin.

A1.1   A. **True.**
       B. **False.**   The PT does not measure contact activation.
       C. **True.**
       D. **True.**
       E. **False.**   No test which takes clot formation as its
                            end-point will detect deficiency of XIII.

Suggested Reading
Hall and Malia, Chapter 15, Basic principles of
haemostatic testing.

A1.2   A. **False.**   Haemoglobin accounts for about 65% of
                          body iron.
       B. **False.**   In health, about 25% of body iron is in the
                          storage form.
       C. **True.**   Myoglobin is a haem-containing substance which
                          acts as an oxygen store for muscles.
       D. **True.**   The normal adult carries up to 3-4 mg of iron
                          bound to plasma transferrin.
       E. **False.**   Total body iron amounts to 3-4 g.

Suggested Reading
Hall and Malia, Chapter 2, Physiology of the blood.

A1.3   A. **False.**   Dietary deficiency of vitamin B_{12} is uncommon
                          in the UK. The commonest cause is PA.
       B. **True.**
       C. **False.**   It is absorbed maximally from the terminal
                          ileum via specific mucosal receptors.
       D. **False.**   Vitamin B_{12} is absent from vegetables.
       E. **False.**   Megaloblastic anaemias typically are macrocytic.

Suggested Reading
Hall and Malia, Chapter 2, Physiology of the blood.

A1.4   A. **False.**   Alanine is not involved in haem synthesis.
       B. **True.**
       C. **False.**   Stercobilin is a breakdown product of
                          haemoglobin.
       D. **True.**
       E. **False.**   Bilirubin is a breakdown product of
                          haemoglobin.

Suggested Reading
Hall and Malia, Chapter 2, Physiology of the blood.

Q1.5 Unincubated osmotic fragility characteristically is increased in the following conditions:

A. hereditary spherocytosis (HS).
B. severe iron deficiency.
C. homozygous haemoglobin C disease.
D. haemolytic disease of the newborn (HDN) due to ABO incompatibility.
E. homozygous β^o thalassaemia.

Q1.6 Haemophilia A (VIII$_c$ deficiency)

A. is inherited as an autosomal dominant character.
B. is characterised by recurrent epistaxis and menorrhagia.
C. is the most common inherited coagulation factor deficiency in the United Kingdom.
D. is characterised by markedly reduced ristocetin cofactor (ricof) activity.
E. is characterised by a prolonged template bleeding time.

Q1.7 The following haemolytic anaemias are caused by extracellular mechanisms:

A. "march" haemoglobinuria.
B. hereditary elliptocytosis (HE).
C. haemolytic disease of the newborn (HDN).
D. paroxysmal nocturnal haemoglobinuria (PNH).
E. favism.

Q1.8 The following conditions predispose strongly to venous thrombosis:

A. antithrombin III (ATIII) deficiency.
B. plasminogen activator inhibitor 1 (PAI-1) deficiency.
C. protein S deficiency.
D. a raised level of heparin cofactor II (HCII).
E. lupus anticoagulant.

A1.5 A. **True.** Spherocytes cannot absorb as much water as normal red cells before bursting.

  B. **False.** Microcytes are capable of absorbing more water than normal red cells before bursting.

  C. **False.** Target cells are resistant to lysis.

  D. **True.** See A

  E. **False.** See B.

Suggested Reading
Chanarin, Chapter 5, Haemolytic anaemia.

A1.6 A. **False.** Haemophilia A is an X-linked recessive disorder.

  B. **False.** It is characterised by haematomata and haemarthroses.

  C. **True.** It has a total incidence in the UK of 5-10/10,000.

  D. **False.** This is suggestive of von Willebrand's disease.

  E. **False.** The bleeding time is a measure of primary haemostasis and is usually normal.

Suggested Reading
Hall and Malia, Chapter 16, Haemorrhagic disorders.

A1.7 A. **True.** March haemoglobinuria is caused by repeated mechanical trauma to the hands or feet.

  B. **False.** HE is caused by an abnormality of the red cell cytoskeleton.

  C. **True.** HDN is antibody-mediated.

  D. **False.** PNH is caused by a membrane defect.

  E. **False.** Favism is associated with G-6-PD deficiency.

Suggested Reading
Hall and Malia, Chapter 11, Haemolytic anaemias.

A1.8 A. **True.**

  B. **False.** PAI-1 is an inhibitor of fibrinolysis. An *excess* predisposes to venous thrombosis.

  C. **True.**

  D. **False.** HCII is a specific inhibitor of thrombin. *Deficiency* predisposes to venous thrombosis.

  E. **True.**

Suggested Reading
Hall and Malia, Chapter 2, Physiology of the blood.

Q1.9 Primary acquired sideroblastic anaemia

A. typically presents in infancy.
B. is characterised by severe microcytosis.
C. can almost always be treated successfully with vitamin B_6.
D. is characterised by the presence of at least 15% ring sideroblasts in the bone marrow.
E. is characterised by marked ineffective erythropoiesis.

Q1.10 The following statements relate to pernicious anaemia (PA):

A. antibodies against gastric parietal cells are found in the serum of 85-90% of patients.
B. type I antibodies prevent vitamin B_{12} from binding to intrinsic factor.
C. type II antibodies are only seen if type I antibodies are also present.
D. up to 80% of cases have neither type I nor type II antibody in their serum.
E. The intrinsic factor and parietal cell antibodies are almost always IgM.

Q1.11 The following are haemoglobin M's:

A. haemoglobin Boston.
B. haemoglobin Lepore.
C. haemoglobin Zürich.
D. haemoglobin Iwate.
E. haemoglobin Milwaukee.

Q1.12 The following features are characteristic of hereditary spherocytosis (HS):

A. autosomal recessive inheritance.
B. deficiency of the red cell cytoskeletal protein ankyrin.
C. increased activity of the red cell cation pump.
D. spherocytic reticulocytes.
E. increased red cell membrane lipid content.

A1.9 A. **False.** Primary acquired sideroblastic anaemia is mainly a disease of the elderly.
       B. **False.** The blood picture typically is macrocytic with anisocytosis and poikilocytosis.
       C. **False.** About 30% of cases show some response to pyridoxine, but in the majority of these only a partial response is obtained.
       D. **True.** Typically, 20-80% ring sideroblasts are present.
       E. **True.**

Suggested Reading
Hall and Malia, Chapter 12, Refractory anaemias.

A1.10 A. **True.** The presence of anti-parietal cell antibodies is characteristic but not diagnostic.
       B. **True.**
       C. **True.**
       D. **False.** Typically, about 75% of cases express type I antibody and 50% have type II antibody.
       E. **False.** The antibodies are mostly IgG or IgA.

Suggested Reading
Hall and Malia, Chapter 10 Macrocytosis and the megaloblastic anaemias.

A1.11 A. **True.** Hb Boston is denoted $\alpha 58(E7)$ his–>tyr.
       B. **False.** Hb Lepore is a $\delta\beta$ chain fusion variant.
       C. **False.** Hb Zürich is an unstable haemoglobin and is denoted $\beta 63(E3)$ his–>arg.
       D. **True.** Hb Iwate is denoted $\alpha 87(F8)$ tyr–>his.
       E. **True.** Hb Milwaukee is denoted $\beta 67(E7)$ val–>glu.

Suggested Reading
Hall and Malia, Chapter 11, Haemolytic anaemias.

A1.12 A. **False.** HS is an autosomal dominant condition.
       B. **False.** The cytoskeletal protein spectrin is deficient or defective in HS.
       C. **True.** This is required to clear excess sodium ions which the defective membrane admits.
       D. **False.** Sphering occurs with increasing red cell age.
       E. **False.** Membrane lipid is lost during sphering.

Suggested Reading
Hall and Malia, Chapter 11, Haemolytic anaemias.

Q1.13 Prothrombin (factor II)

A. is converted to thrombin by the action of Taipan
(*Oxyuranus scuttelatus*) venom.
B. contains serine at its active site.
C. exists as a two-chain molecule linked by disulphide bonds.
D. is converted to thrombin by ancrod (Arvin).
E. levels can fall to 5% without failure of haemostasis.

**Q1.14 The following immunoglobulins strongly activate
Complement via the Classical pathway:**

A. IgD.
B. IgG_2.
C. IgM.
D. IgG_1.
E. IgA.

**Q1.15 Haemoglobin F levels typically are raised in the following
conditions:**

A. homozygous β^+ thalassaemia in a 6-year-old child.
B. Fanconi's anaemia.
C. juvenile chronic myeloid leukaemia (CML).
D. haemoglobin H disease.
E. heterozygous γ thalassaemia in a 6-week-old child.

**Q1.16 The following laboratory results are characteristic of
typical cases of hairy cell leukaemia:**

A. staining for β glucuronidase activity negative.
B. staining for acid phosphatase activity in the presence of
tartrate positive.
C. formation of rosettes with sheep erythrocytes (E-rosettes).
D. staining for α naphthyl butyrate esterase positive with
characteristic crescent pattern.
E. staining for Ia antigen positive.

A1.13 A. **True.** Taipan venom activates prothrombin directly in the presence of phospholipid.
B. **True.** Prothrombin is a serine protease.
C. **False.** Prothrombin is a single chain molecule.
D. **False.** This snake (*Agkistrodon rhodostoma*) venom attacks fibrinogen.
E. **False.** The minimum level required for haemostasis is 40-50%.

Suggested Reading
Hall and Malia, Chapter 2, Physiology of the blood.

A1.14 A. **False.** IgD does not activate Complement.
B. **False.** IgG_2 activates this pathway very weakly.
C. **True.**
D. **True.**
E. **False.** IgA activates the Alternative pathway.

Suggested Reading
Hoffbrand and Lewis, Chapter 8, Blood group serology.

A1.15 A. **True.**
B. **True.**
C. **True.**
D. **False.** HbH disease is a form of α thalassaemia. The HbF is reduced.
E. **False.** HbF ($\alpha_2\gamma_2$) is reduced in γ thalassaemia.

Suggested Reading
Eastham, Chapter 1, Haemoglobin and associated pigments.

A1.16 A. **True.** β glucuronidase is a T cell marker. T-HCL is rare.
B. **True.** This is characteristic, but not diagnostic of hairy cell leukaemia.
C. **False.** This is a marker of T cells.
D. **True.**
E. **True.** Ia is demonstrable on most blood cells except T cells.

Suggested Reading
Hall and Malia, Chapter 13, The proliferative disorders.

Q1.17 The following features are characteristic of congenital dyserythropoietic anaemia (CDA) type II (HEMPAS):

A. autosomal recessive inheritance.
B. a positive Ham's acidified serum test.
C. strong agglutination of the red cells by anti-i.
D. haemolysis induced by incubation of patient red cells with most normal adult sera.
E. at least 15% ring sideroblasts in the bone marrow.

Q1.18 Neutrophil function characteristically is defective in the following conditions:

A. chronic granulomatous disease (CGD).
B. Schwachman's syndrome.
C. Job's syndrome.
D. Chediak-Higashi-Steinbrinck syndrome.
E. Blackfan-Diamond syndrome.

Q1.19 The following features are recognised as indicators of poor prognosis in childhood acute lymphoblastic leukaemia (ALL) if present at diagnosis:

A. female patient.
B. L3 morphology in the bone marrow.
C. common ALL phenotype (ie cALLA-positive).
D. mediastinal mass.
E. white cell count greater than 50×10^9/l.

Q1.20 The following substances are recognised inhibitors of platelet function *in vivo*.

A. sulphinpyrazone.
B. dipyridamole.
C. thromboxane A_2 (TXA$_2$).
D. prostaglandin I_2 (PGI$_2$).
E. ristocetin.

A1.17 A. **True.**

B. **True.** This rare condition differs from PNH, however, in that the patient's own acidified serum does not induce haemolysis.

C. **True.**

D. **False.** HEMPAS red cells are lysed by no more than 30% of normal adult sera.

E. **False.** Ring sideroblasts are not a feature of this disease.

Suggested Reading
Hall and Malia, Chapter 12, Refractory anaemias.

A1.18 A. **True.**

B. **True.**

C. **True.**

D. **True.**

E. **False.** This is pure red cell aplasia.

Suggested Reading
Hoffbrand and Lewis, Chapter 11, Granulocytes, monocytes and their benign disorders.

A1.19 A. **False.** Boys have a rather poorer prognosis because of the possibility of testicular relapse.

B. **True.** This is associated with B-ALL and has a very poor prognosis.

C. **False.** CD10 (cALLA-) positive cases have a much better prognosis than CD10 negative cases.

D. **True.** This is associated with T-ALL and a poor prognosis.

E. **True.**

Suggested Reading
Hall and Malia, Chapter 13, The proliferative disorders.

A1.20 A. **True.** Sulphinpyrazone acts as a competitive inhibitor of cyclo-oxygenase.

B. **True.** Dipyridamole inhibits phosphodiesterase, leading to an increased cAMP level.

C. **False.** TXA_2 is a potent aggregating agent.

D. **True.** PGI_2 inhibits platelet adhesion and aggregation.

E. **False.**

Suggested Reading
Eastham, Chapter 6, Bleeding, clotting and transfusion.

Multiple Choice Test Two

Q2.1 **The following conditions are inherited as autosomal dominant characters:**

A. haemophilia A (VIII_c deficiency).
B. type I von Willebrand's disease.
C. prothrombin (factor II) deficiency.
D. Bernard-Soulier syndrome.
E. factor XIII deficiency.

Q2.2 **The absolute neutrophil count typically increases in response to**

A. prolonged strenuous exercise.
B. deficiency of vitamin B_{12}.
C. large doses of steroid drugs eg prednisone.
D. effective treatment with the drug 6-mercaptopurine.
E. exposure to large doses of X-rays.

Q2.3 **The mature red cell in a normal adult**

A. has a mean surface area of 140 μm^2.
B. has a mean diameter on fixed films of 7.2 μm.
C. has a mean life-span in the circulation of 120 days.
D. has clumped nuclear chromatin.
E. is spherical in shape.

Q2.4 **The following coagulation factors are activated directly by thrombin:**

A. factor V.
B. factor VIII_c.
C. factor XIII.
D. factor XI.
E. factor I (fibrinogen).

A2.1 A. **False.** Haemophilia A is an X-linked recessive disorder.
  B. **True.**
  C. **False.** Prothrombin deficiency is an autosomal recessive disorder.
  D. **False.** Bernard-Soulier syndrome is an autosomal recessive disorder.
  E. **False.** Factor XIII deficiency is an autosomal recessive disorder.

Suggested Reading
  Hall and Malia, Chapter 16, Haemorrhagic disorders.

A2.2 A. **True.** Strenuous exercise induces release of neutrophils from the marginated pool.
  B. **False.** Vitamin B_{12} deficiency is associated with pancytopenia.
  C. **True.** Steroids decrease the rate at which neutrophils leave the circulation.
  D. **False.** 6-MP is a cytoreductive agent.
  E. **False.** X-rays damage stem cells and may cause aplasia.

Suggested Reading
  Eastham, Chapter 4, Peripheral white blood cells.

A2.3 A. **True.**
  B. **True.**
  C. **True.**
  D. **False.** Mature red cells have no nucleus.
  E. **False.** Normal red cells are biconcave discs.

Suggested Reading
  Hall and Malia, Chapter 2, Physiology of the blood.

A2.4 A. **True.**
  B. **True.**
  C. **True.**
  D. **False.**
  E. **True.**

Suggested Reading
  Hall and Malia, Chapter 2, Physiology of the blood.

Q2.5 The following values are normal for a 70 kg adult male:

A. an absolute monocyte count of 0.6×10^9/l.
B. an absolute reticulocyte count of 450×10^9/l.
C. a venous haematocrit of 0.55.
D. an active bone marrow volume of 2.0 litres.
E. a plasma volume of 3.0 litres.

Q2.6 A normal 6-week-old embryo is synthesising the following haemoglobins or haemoglobin precursors:

A. haemoglobin Gower I ($\zeta_2\varepsilon_2$).
B. δ globin chains.
C. α globin chains.
D. β globin chains.
E. haemoglobin Portland ($\zeta_2\gamma_2$).

Q2.7 The following reagents will correct a prolonged prothrombin time due to factor VII deficiency:

A. aluminium hydroxide adsorbed plasma.
B. aged serum.
C. barium sulphate eluate.
D. aged oxalated plasma.
E. normal plasma.

Q2.8 The following conditions predispose strongly to vitamin B_{12} deficiency in the absence of prophylaxis:

A. total gastrectomy.
B. successful methotrexate therapy.
C. Imerslund-Gräsbeck syndrome.
D. infestation with the fish tapeworm *Diphyllobothrium latum*.
E. diverticulitis of the small bowel.

A2.5 A. **True.** The normal range for absolute monocyte count is $0.2-0.8 \times 10^9/l$.
 B. **False.** The normal range for absolute reticulocyte count is $20-100 \times 10^9/l$.
 C. **False.** The normal range for PCV is 0.40-0.52.
 D. **True.** Adults have 4 litres of bone marrow of which about 50% is haemopoietically active.
 E. **True.** Normal plasma volume is 40-50 ml/kg.

Suggested Reading
Eastham, Chapters 1, 2 and 5.

A2.6 A. **True.** Hb Gower I is synthesised until 10/40.
 B. **False.** δ globin is not synthesised until about 30/40.
 C. **True.** α globin is detectable at about 5/40.
 D. **False.** β globin synthesis does not begin until 10/40.
 E. **True.** Hb Portland is synthesised until 10/40.

Suggested Reading
Hall and Malia, Chapter 2, Physiology of the blood.

A2.7 A. **False.** This reagent is deficient in factors II, VII, IX and X.
 B. **True.** This reagent contains factors VII, IX, X, XI and XII.
 C. **True.** This reagent contains factors II, VII, IX and X.
 D. **True.** This reagent contains all factors except V.
 E. **True.**

Suggested Reading
Hall and Malia, Chapter 15, Basic principles of haemostatic testing.

A2.8 A. **True.** Gastrectomy removes the source of IF.
 B. **False.** Methotrexate inhibits folate metabolism.
 C. **True.** This inherited condition is manifest as selective malabsorption of vitamin B_{12} with proteinuria.
 D. **True.** The parasites compete successfully for dietary vitamin B_{12}.
 E. **True.** Bacterial overgrowth in the diverticula results in increased competition for dietary vitamin B_{12}.

Suggested Reading
Hoffbrand and Lewis, Chapter 3, Megaloblastic anaemias.

Q2.9 **The plasma haemoglobin level typically is increased in the following conditions:**

A. hereditary spherocytosis (HS).
B. homozygous β^o thalassaemia.
C. paroxysmal nocturnal haemoglobinuria (PNH).
D. blackwater fever (associated with *Plasmodium falciparum* malaria).
E. after an ABO-incompatible blood transfusion.

Q2.10 **The following laboratory results are consistent with a diagnosis of heterozygous β^+ thalassaemia in an adult female:**

A. a haemoglobin A_2 level of 4.8%.
B. an $\alpha{:}\beta$ globin chain synthesis ratio of 0.8.
C. a reduced red cell osmotic fragility.
D. a RBC of 4.33 x 10^{12}/l, a Hb of 9.2 g/dl and an MCV of 63 fl.
E. mild microcytic, hypochromic anaemia with target cells on the blood film.

Q2.11 **The following reagents are required in the ICSH recommended (Betke's) technique for the quantitation of haemoglobin F:**

A. Drabkin's solution.
B. 0.2M hydrochloric acid.
C. saturated ammonium sulphate solution.
D. veronal buffer.
E. dithiothreitol (DTT).

Q2.12 **Thrombocytopenia typically is present in the following conditions:**

A. Henoch Schönlein purpura.
B. Grey platelet syndrome.
C. Bernard-Soulier syndrome.
D. Wiskott-Aldrich syndrome.
E. May-Hegglin anomaly.

A2.9   A. **False.**   Haemolysis is mainly extravascular in HS.
       B. **True.**   Plasma haemoglobin is increased where intravascular haemolysis has recently taken place.
       C. **True.**
       D. **True.**
       E. **True.**

Suggested Reading
Hall and Malia, Chapter 11, Haemolytic anaemia.

A2.10   A. **True.**
       B. **False.**   The $\alpha{:}\beta$ synthesis ratio typically is greater than 1.5 in β^+ thalassaemia heterozygotes.
       C. **True.**
       D. **False.**   These values produce a positive result for the discriminant function (MCV-(5xHb)-RBC-6.8).
       E. **True.**   This appearance is characteristic.

Suggested Reading
Hall and Malia, Chapter 9, Microcytic anaemias.

A2.11   A. **True.**
       B. **False.**   The method is based on the resistance of HbF to alkali denaturation.
       C. **True.**   This is used as a precipitating agent.
       D. **False.**
       E. **False.**   DTT is a reducing agent used in the assay of folate.

Suggested Reading
Chanarin, Chapter 2, Haemoglobin analysis.

A2.12   A. **False.**   Henoch-Schönlein purpura is a vasculopathy.
       B. **True.**
       C. **True.**
       D. **True.**
       E. **True.**

Suggested Reading
Hall and Malia, Chapter 16, Haemorrhagic disorders.

Q2.13 **Heinz bodies**

A. consist of denatured globin.
B. can be induced in normal red cells by exposure to acetanilide.
C. are a recognised feature of glucose-6-phosphate dehydrogenase (G-6-PD) deficiency.
D. lead to a shortened red cell survival.
E. are a recognised feature of haemoglobin Köln disease.

Q2.14 **The following laboratory results are consistent with a diagnosis of aplastic anaemia:**

A. a leucocyte alkaline phosphatase (LAP) score of 11/100 neutrophils.
B. a raised level of haemoglobin F.
C. a reduced number of CFU-GM in *in-vitro* cell culture.
D. the presence of the chromosomal translocation t(9q+;22q-).
E. an absolute reticulocyte count of 50 x 10^9/l in an adult female.

Q2.15 **The following statements relate to the coagulation inhibitor antithrombin III (ATIII):**

A. predisposition to myocardial infarction (MI) is a typical feature of ATIII deficiency.
B. it exists as a two-chain molecule linked by disulphide bridges.
C. it has a molecular weight of 58,000 daltons.
D. homozygous AT III deficiency is the commonest hereditary condition which predisposes to thrombosis.
E. the minimum circulating level for effective antithrombotic activity is about 10%.

Q2.16 **The following features are characteristic of the blasts of L1 acute leukaemia:**

A. a high nuclear:cytoplasmic ratio.
B. one inconspicuous nucleolus.
C. intense cytoplasmic basophilia.
D. prominent cytoplasmic vacuolation.
E. Sudan black staining negative.

21

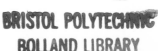

A2.13 A. **True.**
B. **True.**
C. **True.** Heinz bodies are most commonly seen in drug-induced haemolysis.
D. **True.** Heinz bodies are removed by the spleen.
E. **True.** Hb Köln is an unstable haemoglobin.

Suggested Reading
Hall and Malia, Chapter 11, Haemolytic anaemias.

A2.14 A. **False.** LAP typically is increased in aplastic anaemia. The normal range is 15-100.
B. **True.**
C. **True.**
D. **False.** This is the Philadelphia chromosome which is characteristic of CML.
E. **False.** Reticulocytopenia is present in aplastic anaemia. The normal range is 20-100 x 10^9/l.

Suggested Reading
Hoffbrand and Lewis, Chapter 4, Aplastic anaemia and other types of bone marrow failure.

A2.15 A. **False.** There is no predisposition to arterial thrombosis in ATIII deficiency.
B. **False.** ATIII is a single chain molecule.
C. **True.**
D. **False.** Homozygous ATIII deficiency has not been described and is probably incompatible with life.
E. **False.** An excess of venous thrombosis is observed if the ATIII level falls below about 70%.

Suggested Reading
Hoffbrand and Lewis, Chapter 21, Normal haemostasis.

A2.16 A. **True.** L1 blasts typically have scanty cytoplasm.
B. **True.**
C. **False.** This is characteristic of L3.
D. **False.** This is characteristic of L3.
E. **True.**

Suggested Reading
Hall and Malia, Chapter 13, The proliferative disorders.

Q2.17 **Platelet α granules contain the following substances:**

A. platelet factor 4 (anti-heparin factor).
B. 5-hydroxytryptamine (serotonin).
C. fibronectin.
D. β-thromboglobulin.
E. coagulation factor V.

Q2.18 **A normal reticulocyte has the following metabolic capabilities:**

A. DNA synthesis.
B. haem synthesis.
C. tricarboxylic acid cycle (Krebs' cycle).
D. anaerobic glycolytic activity.
E. RNA synthesis.

Q2.19 **The following statements relate to the electrophoretic mobilities of haemoglobin variants at pH 8.4:**

A. haemoglobin S does not separate from haemoglobin G.
B. haemoglobin D migrates towards the anode.
C. haemoglobin H migrates more rapidly than haemoglobin A.
D. haemoglobins D and E do not separate.
E. haemoglobin F migrates more rapidly than haemoglobin A.

Q2.20 **5,10-methylene tetrahydrofolate**

A. acts as a co-enzyme of thymidylate synthetase in the conversion of deoxyuridylate (dUMP) to deoxythymidylate (dTMP).
B. is converted to tetrahydrofolate during the conversion of dUMP to dTMP.
C. acts as a cofactor in the methylation of homocysteine to methionine.
D. is derived from tetrahydrofolate which acts as a co-factor in the conversion of serine to glycine.
E. is destroyed by the administration of nitrous oxide, thus leading to megaloblastosis.

A2.17 A. True.
      B. False.   Serotonin is a constituent of dense granules.
      C. True.
      D. True.
      E. True.

Suggested Reading
Hoffbrand and Lewis, Chapter 21, Normal haemostasis.

A2.18 A. False.   Reticulocytes have no nucleus.
      B. True.   The few residual mitochondria are capable of maintaining haem synthesis.
      C. True.   The Krebs' cycle occurs in mitochondria.
      D. True.   The EM pathway remains intact, even in the mature red cell.
      E. False.   Reticulocytes have no nucleus.

Suggested Reading
Hoffbrand and Lewis, Chapter 6, Inherited haemolytic anaemias.

A2.19 A. True.
      B. True.
      C. True.
      D. False.   HbE migrates more slowly than HbD.
      E. False.

Suggested Reading
Chanarin, Chapter 2, Haemoglobin analysis.

A2.20 A. True.
      B. False.   5,10-methylene THF is converted to dihydrofolate.
      C. False.   5-methyl THF acts as a cofactor in the methylation of homocysteine.
      D. True.
      E. False.   Nitrous oxide induces megaloblastosis by inactivation of vitamin B_{12}.

Suggested Reading
Hall and Malia, Chapter 10, Macrocytosis and the megaloblastic anaemias.

Multiple Choice Test Three

Q3.1 The following statements relate to abnormalities of red cell morphology:

A. schistocytes are fragmented red cells.
B. acanthocytes are regularly-shaped oval red cells.
C. leptocytes are also known as "target" cells.
D. stomatocytes are shaped like teardrops.
E. drepanocytes are most commonly seen in alcoholic liver disease.

Q3.2 The following statements relate to the coagulation factor VIII_c:

A. the gene which codes for VIII_c is present on chromosome 16.
B. it is markedly deficient in Christmas disease.
C. its functional activity is measured using the ristocetin cofactor (ricof) assay.
D. it is not consumed during coagulation.
E. it is a vitamin K-dependent coagulation factor.

Q3.3 The number of megakaryocytes in a bone marrow smear characteristically is decreased in the following conditions:

A. decompensated disseminated intravascular coagulation (DIC).
B. untreated pernicious anaemia (PA).
C. thrombotic thrombocytopenic purpura (TTP).
D. idiopathic thrombocytopenic purpura (ITP).
E. polycythaemia rubra vera (PRV).

A3.1   A. **True.**
         B. **False.**   Acanthocytes are irregularly shaped cells with spiny projections.
         C. **True.**
         D. **False.**   Stomatocytes are characterised by a slit-like area of central pallor.
         E. **False.**   Drepanocytes are sickle cells.

Suggested Reading
Hall and Malia, Chapter 5, Preparation, staining and examination of blood films.

A3.2   A. **False.** VIII_c is coded for on the X chromosome.
         B. **False.**   Factor IX is deficient in Christmas disease.
         C. **False.**   The ricof assay measures the ability of vWF to induce platelet aggregation in the presence of ristocetin.
         D. **False.**
         E. **False.**

Suggested Reading
Hall and Malia, Chapter 2, Physiology of the blood.

A3.3   A. **False.**   Thrombocytopenia in DIC is a result of consumption, not failure of production.
         B. **True.**
         C. **False.**   TTP is characterised by platelet consumption.
         D. **False.**   ITP is characterised by antibody-mediated destruction of platelets.
         E. **False.**   Megakaryocyte numbers typically are normal or increased in PRV.

Suggested Reading
Hoffbrand and Lewis, Chapter 22, Platelet disorders.

Q3.4 **The following statements relate to the action and laboratory control of oral anticoagulants such as warfarin:**

A. they prevent the synthesis of coagulation factors II, VII, IX and X.
B. the first factor to be reduced in activity by their action is prothrombin (factor II).
C. the international normalised ratio (INR) is derived using the formula INR = prothrombin time ratio (PTR) x international sensitivity index (ISI).
D. anticoagulation is complete within 1 h of ingestion.
E. they cross the placental barrier and can cause foetal haemorrhage.

Q3.5 **The following statements relate to normal lymphocytes:**

A. at least 75% of peripheral blood lymphocytes are B cells.
B. the membranes of mature B lymphocytes carry surface immunoglobulin (SIg).
C. γ intèrferon is synthesised by B lymphocytes.
D. B lymphocytes spontaneously form rosettes with sheep red cells (E-rosettes).
E. graft versus host disease (GVHD) is mediated by B lymphocytes.

Q3.6 **The following statements relate to normal globins:**

A. ζ globin contains 141 amino acid residues.
B. δ chain synthesis ceases just before birth.
C. α chains contain no histidyl residues.
D. γ chains contain 122 amino acid residues.
E. the genes for globin chain synthesis all reside on chromosome 11.

A3.4   A. **False.** Warfarin blocks the post-translational γ-carboxylation of the vitamin K-dependent factors. Synthesis is not reduced.

       B. **False.** The level of factor VII falls first because it has the shortest biological half-life.

       C. **False.** INR = PTR^{ISI}

       D. **False.** Full anticoagulation takes about 60 h although factor VII activity falls within 6 h.

       E. **True.**

Suggested Reading
Hall and Malia, Chapter 17, Thrombosis.

A3.5   A. **False.** About 10-15% of peripheral blood lymphocytes are B cells.

       B. **True.**

       C. **False.** γ interferon is synthesised by T cells.

       D. **False.** E-rosette formation is a T cell marker.

       E. **False.** GVHD is mediated by T cells.

Suggested Reading
Hall and Malia, Chapter 2, Physiology of the blood.

A3.6   A. **True.** ζ globin is the embryonic form of α globin.

       B. **False.** δ globin synthesis continues into adulthood.

       C. **False.** Haem is bound to the globin chain via histidyl residues.

       D. **False.** γ globin contains 146 amino acid residues.

       E. **False.** The α globin gene cluster resides on chromosome 16, and the β globin gene cluster resides on chromosome 11.

Suggested Reading
Hall and Malia, Chapter 1, Haemopoiesis.

Q3.7 Haemolysis is primarily intravascular in the following conditions:

A. hereditary spherocytosis (HS).
B. *Clostridium welchii* (*C. perfringens*) septicaemia.
C. paroxysmal nocturnal haemoglobinuria (PNH).
D. favism.
E. after ABO-incompatible blood transfusion.

Q3.8 The following statements relate to the plasma transport of vitamin B_{12}:

A. the main plasma transport form is hydroxycobalamin.
B. transcobalamin I is synthesised by granulocytes.
C. transcobalamin II is normally 70-80% saturated with vitamin B_{12}.
D. transcobalamin I acts as a reserve store of vitamin B_{12} because of its high avidity for methylcobalamin.
E. most intracellular vitamin B_{12} is in the form of methylcobalamin.

Q3.9 The following statements relate to the cell cycle:

A. cells in G_2 phase are tetraploid.
B. cells in G_0 are about to divide.
C. the proportion of cells in S phase can be measured by their ability to utilise tritiated thymidine.
D. cells at the completion of S phase are diploid.
E. mitosis immediately precedes G_2 phase.

Q3.10 The following features are characteristic of pyruvate kinase (PK) deficiency:

A. marked spherocytosis on the blood film.
B. neonatal jaundice.
C. X-linked recessive inheritance.
D. acute haemolysis precipitated by exposure to fava beans.
E. the anaemia is poorly tolerated due to accumulation of 2,3-diphosphoglycerate (2,3-DPG) in the red cells.

A3.7   A. **False.** The main site of haemolysis in HS is the spleen.
          B. **True.**
          C. **True.**
          D. **True.**
          E. **True.**

Suggested Reading
Hall and Malia, Chapter 11, Haemolytic anaemias.

A3.8   A. **False.** The major plasma form of vitamin B_{12} is methylcobalamin.
          B. **True.** This explains the markedly raised serum vitamin B_{12} levels seen in CML.
          C. **False.** TCII is normally less than 5% saturated.
          D. **True.**
          E. **False.** 70-80% of intracellular vitamin B_{12} is in the form of $5'$-deoxyadenosylcobalamin.

Suggested Reading
Hall and Malia, Chapter 10, Macrocytosis and the megaloblastic anaemias.

A3.9   A. **True.** G_2 is immediately before mitosis.
          B. **False.** G_0 cells are "resting".
          C. **True.**
          D. **False.** They are tetraploid.
          E. **False.**

Suggested Reading
Hall and Malia, Chapter 1, Haemopoiesis.

A3.10 A. **False.** PK deficiency typically is a CNSHA.
          B. **True.** Neonatal jaundice may be severe enough to require exchange transfusion.
          C. **False.** This is an autosomal recessive condition.
          D. **False.** This is a feature of G-6-PD deficiency.
          E. **False.** Increased 2,3-DPG leads to improved tolerance of the anaemia.

Suggested Reading
Hall and Malia, Chapter 11, Haemolytic anaemias.

Q3.11 **The following statements relate to the coagulation factor thrombin:**

A. it acts on fibrinogen by cleaving valine-glutamine bonds.
B. it is cleaved into two inactive peptides by antithrombin III (ATIII).
C. it releases fibrinopeptides from the β and γ chains of fibrinogen respectively.
D. it activates factor XIII directly.
E. it combines with thrombomodulin and activates protein C.

Q3.12 **The following changes normally occur as a mature circulating red cell ages:**

A. a gradual accumulation of intracellular potassium.
B. an increase in osmotic fragility.
C. loss of intracellular water.
D. a rise in the MCHC.
E. a decrease in deformability.

Q3.13 **Coagulation factor V**

A. has a molecular weight of 55,000 daltons.
B. is present in platelet α granules.
C. is labile on storage in oxalate as anticoagulant.
D. is synthesised by hepatocytes.
E. is vitamin K-dependent.

Q3.14 **The following laboratory results are consistent with a diagnosis of α thalassaemia-1 trait (α-/α- or $\alpha\alpha$/--):**

A. 10% haemoglobin Barts in the cord blood.
B. raised levels of haemoglobins A_2 and F in an adult.
C. an α:β globin chain synthesis ratio of 1.8.
D. a microcytic, hypochromic blood picture.
E. 5% haemoglobin Portland in a 3-week-old child.

A3.11 A. **False.** Thrombin cleaves arginine-lysine bonds.
B. **False.** ATIII combines irreversibly with thrombin, rendering it inactive.
C. **False.** Fibrinopeptides A and B are released from the α and β chains respectively.
D. **True.**
E. **True.**

Suggested Reading
Hoffbrand and Lewis, Chapter 21, Normal haemostasis.

A3.12 A. **False.** Activity of the EM pathway decreases as the red cell ages, leading to failure of the cation pump, loss of K^+ and water. This results in increased osmotic fragility and a higher MCHC.
B. **True.**
C. **True.**
D. **True.**
E. **True.**

Suggested Reading
Hoffbrand and Lewis, Chapter 6, Inherited haemolytic anaemias.

A3.13 A. **False.** Factor V has a molecular weight of 330,000-350,000 daltons.
B. **True.**
C. **True.** This is exploited in the preparation of factor V-deficient plasma by ageing.
D. **True.**
E. **False.**

Suggested Reading
Hoffbrand and Lewis, Chapter 21, Normal haemostasis.

A3.14 A. **True.**
B. **False.** This would be suggestive of β thalassaemia.
C. **False.** The α:β synthesis ratio is <1.0 in α thalassaemia.
D. **True.**
E. **False.** Hb Portland is only synthesised up to 10 weeks gestation.

Suggested Reading
Hall and Malia, Chapter 9, Microcytic anaemias.

Q3.15 The following laboratory results are characteristic of the blast cells of pre-B acute lymphoblastic leukaemia (ALL):

A. cytoplasmic IgM (CIg) demonstrable by immunofluorescence.
B. staining for terminal deoxynucleotidyl transferase (TdT) positive.
C. formation of rosettes with sheep erythrocytes (E-rosettes).
D. surface immunoglobulin (SIg) demonstrable by immunofluorescence.
E. staining for Ia antigen positive.

Q3.16 Chronic granulomatous disease (CGD)

A. typically is inherited as an X-linked recessive disorder.
B. is characterised by recurrent infections with organisms such as *Staphylococcus aureus*.
C. is characterised by severe neutropenia.
D. is caused by deficiency of the enzyme superoxide dismutase (SOD).
E. is characterised by failure of the neutrophils to convert nitroblue tetrazolium to formazan.

Q3.17 The following statements relate to the Schilling test of vitamin B_{12} absorption:

A. falsely normal results may be obtained if collection of urine is incomplete.
B. normal individuals excrete at least 10% of the test dose within 24 h.
C. a "flushing dose" of ^{58}Co-labelled vitamin B_{12} is administered before the test dose.
D. correction of an abnormal result by simultaneous administration of intrinsic factor is consistent with pernicious anaemia (PA).
E. the test dose of radioactive vitamin B_{12} is injected intravenously.

A3.15 A. **True.**

         B. **True.**

         C. **False.** This is a T cell marker.

         D. **False.** Surface immunoglobulin is a marker of mature B cells.

         E. **True.**

Suggested Reading

Hall and Malia, Chapter 13, The proliferative disorders.

A3.16 A. **True.** A very rare autosomal recessive form also exists.

         B. **True.** Infection with Gram-negative organisms and fungi are also troublesome in CGD.

         C. **False.** The absolute neutrophil count typically is normal in CGD.

         D. **False.** CGD is caused by deficiency or a defect of cytochrome b_{245}.

         E. **True.** This forms the basis of the most simple screening test for CGD.

Suggested Reading

Hoffbrand and Lewis, Chapter 11, Granulocytes, monocytes and their benign disorders.

A3.17 A. **False.** Incomplete collection would result in an underestimate of excretion .

         B. **True.** The normal range is 11-32% excretion.

         C. **False.** The flushing dose should be non-radioactive.

         D. **True.**

         E. **False.** The test dose is given orally. The flushing dose is injected intramuscularly.

Suggested Reading

Chanarin, Chapter 6, Megaloblastic anaemias.

Q3.18 **Human IgA immunoglobulin**

A. is the major immunoglobulin present in external body secretions.
B. exists in both monomeric and dimeric forms.
C. mediates the destruction of parasites by eosinophils.
D. does not activate Complement.
E. is present in large amounts in colostrum.

Q3.19 **The following statements relate to haemoglobin S:**

A. the mutation involves the recognition site for the restriction endonuclease Mst II.
B. aplastic crises are a recognised feature of sickle cell disease (HbSS).
C. simultaneous inheritance of homozygous HbS and homozygous α^+ thalassaemia results in an extremely severe anaemia.
D. sickled red cells cannot resume their normal shape.
E. heterozygotes for haemoglobin S are less susceptible to *Plasmodium falciparum* malaria.

Q3.20 **Megaloblastic change in the absence of haematinic deficiency is a recognised feature of the following conditions:**

A. orotic aciduria.
B. effective treatment with the cytotoxic drug 5-Fluorouracil.
C. transcobalamin II (TCII) deficiency.
D. M6 acute leukaemia
E. congenital dyserythropoietic anaemia type II (HEMPAS).

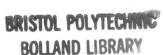

A3.18 A. **True.**
B. **True.** Monomeric IgA is found in the plasma while the dimeric form predominates in body secretions.
C. **False.** Destruction of parasites is the role of IgE.
D. **False.** IgA activates Complement via the alternative pathway.
E. **True.**

Suggested Reading
Hoffbrand and Lewis, Chapter 8, Blood group serology.

A3.19 A. **True.** This enzyme is used in the antenatal diagnosis of sickle cell disease.
B. **True.** Aplastic crises are often associated with infection.
C. **False.** This results in a clinically less severe condition.
D. **False.** Red cells may undergo several sickling episodes before the change is irreversible.
E. **True.**

Suggested Reading
Hoffbrand and Lewis, Chapter 5, The haemoglobinopathies.

A3.20 A. **True.** This rare megaloblastic condition responds to uridine administration.
B. **True.** This antimetabolite interferes with DNA synthesis.
C. **True.** TCII deficiency results in poor delivery of vitamin B_{12} to the bone marrow.
D. **True.**
E. **False.** Nuclear maturation typically is normal in HEMPAS.

Suggested Reading
Hoffbrand and Lewis, Chapter 3, Megaloblastic anaemia.

Multiple Choice Test Four

Q4.1 Drabkin's reagent

    A. contains potassium cyanide.
    B. converts carboxyhaemoglobin to cyanmethaemoglobin.
    C. has a pH of 5.8.
    D. converts sulphaemoglobin to cyanmethaemoglobin.
    E. can be stored at room temperature for several
       months before use.

Q4.2 Normal peripheral blood platelets

    A. have a mean diameter of 2-4 μm.
    B. have a mean volume of 20-30 fl.
    C. survive in the peripheral circulation for 8-11 days.
    D. will aggregate strongly *in vitro* in the presence of ATP.
    E. carry coagulation factor V adsorbed on their surface.

Q4.3 Severe deficiency of the following coagulation
       factors causes prolongation of the APTT:

    A. factor I (fibrinogen).
    B. factor XII.
    C. factor VIII$_c$.
    D. factor VII.
    E. factor XIII.

Q4.4 The following coagulation factors are vitamin K--
       dependent:

    A. factor I (fibrinogen).
    B. protein C.
    C. factor XIII.
    D. factor IX.
    E. factor XI.

A4.1 A. **True.** Drabkin's contains 50 mg/l of KCN.
   B. **True.** All forms of haemoglobin except
            sulphaemoglobin are converted by Drabkin's.
   C. **False.** The pH is 7.0-7.4.
   D. **False.** See B.
   E. **True.**

Suggested Reading
   Chanarin, Chapter 1, The blood count, its quality control
   and related methods.

A4.2 A. **True.**
   B. **False.** The normal MPV is 8-10 fl.
   C. **True.**
   D. **False.** Unlike ADP, ATP is not an aggregating agent.
   E. **True.**

Suggested Reading
   Hall and Malia, Chapter 2, Physiology of the blood.

A4.3 A. **True.** The APTT is a measure of the intrinsic pathway
            and so is sensitive to deficiencies of all
            coagulation factors except VII and XIII.
   B. **True.**
   C. **True.**
   D. **False.**
   E. **False.**

Suggested Reading
   Hall and Malia, Chapter 15, Basic principles of haemostatic
   testing.

A4.4 A. **False.**
   B. **True.**
   C. **False.**
   D. **True.**
   E. **False.**

Suggested Reading
   Hall and Malia, Chapter 2, Physiology of the blood.

Q4.5 The following laboratory results are consistent with a diagnosis of intravascular haemolysis in an adult man:

A. an absolute reticulocyte count of $450 \times 10^9/l$.
B. a positive Schumm's test .
C. haemosiderinuria.
D. haematuria.
E. a raised serum haemopexin level.

Q4.6 The following mechanisms play an important role in innate (non-specific) immunity:

A. phagocytic cells eg neutrophils.
B. natural killer cells.
C. lysozyme.
D. commensal organisms eg the normal gut flora.
E. Complement.

Q4.7 The following statements relate to the FAB classification scheme for acute leukaemia:

A. the microgranular variant of promyelocytic leukaemia is designated M4.
B. acute erythroleukaemia is designated M6.
C. poorly differentiated monoblastic leukaemia is designated M5a.
D. myeloblastic leukaemia with differentiation is designated M3.
E. myeloblastic leukaemia without differentiation is designated M1.

Q4.8 The following findings are characteristic of homozygous α^0 thalassaemia ((--/--), Barts hydrops foetalis):

A. intra-uterine death.
B. 20-30% haemoglobin Portland in the cord blood.
C. a raised haemoglobin A_2 level.
D. ineffective oxygen transport to the tissues.
E. marked erythroblastaemia and anisopoikilocytosis on the blood film.

A4.5   A. **True.**   The normal range is 20-100 x 10^9/l.

        B. **True.**   Schumm's test measures methaemalbumin.

        C. **True.**   Haemosiderinuria is consistent with chronic intravascular haemolysis.

        D. **False.**   Haemoglobinuria is indicative of haemolysis.

        E. **False.**   Serum haemopexin falls in the presence of intravascular haemolysis.

Suggested Reading

Hall and Malia, Chapter 11, Haemolytic anaemia.

A4.6   A. **True.**   Phagocytes form the most important non-specific defence once the skin has been breached.

        B. **False.**   NK cells are an important component of specific immunity.

        C. **True.**   Lysozyme is a bactericidal substance which is present in body secretions.

        D. **True.**   The commensal flora compete with pathogenic organisms for space and nutrients.

        E. **True.**   The Alternative pathway is non-specific.

Suggested Reading

Roitt, Brostoff and Male, Chapter 1, Adaptive and innate immunity.

A4.7   A. **False.**   This is designated M3-variant.

        B. **True.**

        C. **True.**

        D. **False.**   This is M2.

        E. **True.**

Suggested Reading

Hall and Malia, Chapter 13, The proliferative disorders.

A4.8   A. **True.**   Absence of α globin synthesis is incompatible with extra-uterine life.

        B. **True.**   20-30% of the cord blood is Hb Portland ($\zeta_2\gamma_2$), the remainder is Hb Barts (γ_4) and HbH (β_4).

        C. **False.** α globin synthesis is absent.

        D. **True.**   Hb Barts is useless as a respiratory pigment.

        E. **True.**

Suggested Reading

Hall and Malia, Chapter 9, Microcytic anaemias.

Q4.9 The following statements relate to female carriers of haemophilia A:

A. the daughters of a haemophiliac are obligate carriers.
B. a woman whose first child is a haemophiliac is an obligate carrier.
C. they are likely to bleed excessively after minor trauma.
D. most have a VIII_c:vWF ratio greater than 1.2.
E. the daughter of a carrier female and a normal male stands a 1 in 4 chance of being a carrier.

Q4.10 The following statements relate to protein C:

A. its activity is decreased by effective warfarin therapy.
B. activated protein C neutralises activated factor V.
C. its activity requires the presence of calcium ions.
D. it neutralises plasminogen activator inhibitor -1 (PAI-1).
E. it is activated by Russell's viper venom.

Q4.11 The following DNA/RNA bases are purines:

A. adenine.
B. guanine.
C. cytosine.
D. thymine.
E. uracil.

Q4.12 The following laboratory results are characteristic of the myelodysplastic syndrome refractory anaemia (RA):

A. up to 15% ring sideroblasts in the bone marrow.
B. at least 20% blasts in the bone marrow.
C. at least 5% blasts in the peripheral blood.
D. a markedly hypocellular bone marrow.
E. Auer rods common in blasts.

A4.9 A. **True.**
      B. **False.** This could be the result of a spontaneous mutation in the child.
      C. **False.** Carriers typically are symptomless.
      D. **False.** Most have a VIII_c:vWF of less than 0.7.
      E. **False.** The probability is 1 in 2.

Suggested Reading

Hall and Malia, Chapter 16, Haemorrhagic disorders.

A4.10 A. **True.** Protein C is vitamin K-dependent.
       B. **True.**
       C. **True.**
       D. **True.**
       E. **True.**

Suggested Reading

Hoffbrand and Lewis, Chapter 21, Normal haemostasis.

A4.11 A. **True.**
       B. **True.**
       C. **False.** Cytosine is a pyrimidine.
       D. **False.** Thymine is a pyrimidine.
       E. **False.** Uracil is a pyrimidine.

Suggested Reading

Hall and Malia, Chapter 1, Haemopoiesis.

A4.12 A. **True.**
       B. **False.** RA is defined as having less than 5% blasts in the bone marrow.
       C. **False.** This is consistent with RAEB-t.
       D. **False.** The bone marrow is normo- or hypercellular.
       E. **False.** This is consistent with RAEB-t.

Suggested Reading

Hoffbrand and Lewis, Chapter 17, The myelodysplastic syndromes.

Q4.13   The following disorders are characterised by morphological abnormalities of neutrophils recognisable using light microscopy:

A. Pelger-Huët anomaly.
B. May-Hegglin anomaly.
C. Jordan's anomaly.
D. Alder-Reilly anomaly.
E. Undritz anomaly.

Q4.14   The following laboratory results are consistent with a diagnosis of severe megaloblastic anaemia:

A. a positive Schumm's test for methaemalbumin.
B. an increased plasma level of unconjugated bilirubin.
C. increased excretion of urobilinogen in faeces and urine.
D. reduced levels of plasma lactic dehydrogenase (LDH).
E. increased plasma lysozyme levels.

Q4.15   Human IgG immunoglobulin

A. can cross the placental barrier.
B. is concerned mainly with the primary antibody response.
C. accounts for 70-80% of serum immunoglobulins.
D. is composed of at least 75% subclass IgG_2.
E. is capable of precipitating soluble bacterial toxins.

Q4.16   The following features are characteristic of M3 acute leukaemia:

A. bundles (faggots) of Auer rods in the cytoplasm of the leukaemic cells.
B. a monomorphic population of myeloblasts in the bone marrow smear.
C. Sudan black staining negative.
D. terminal deoxynucleotidyl transferase (TdT) staining positive.
E. the presence of disseminated intravascular coagulation (DIC).

A4.13 A. **True.** This autosomal dominant condition is manifest as neutrophil hyposegmentation.
   B. **True.** This condition is characterised by Döhle bodies.
   C. **True.** This condition is characterised by prominent vacuolation of the neutrophils.
   D. **True.** This autosomal recessive condition is characterised by abnormally large granules.
   E. **True.** This autosomal recessive condition is manifest as neutrophil hypersegmentation.

Suggested Reading
Hoffbrand and Lewis, Chapter 11, Granulocytes, monocytes and their benign disorders.

A4.14 A. **True.** This is a reflection of decreased red cell survival and intramedullary cell death.
   B. **True.** This is a reflection of increased haemoglobin catabolism.
   C. **True.** See B.
   D. **False.** Plasma LDH levels are increased.
   E. **True.** This is a reflection of intramedullary death of granulocytes.

Suggested Reading
Hoffbrand and Lewis, Chapter 3, Megaloblastic anaemia.

A4.15 A. **True.** This is the main source of passive immunity in neonates.
   B. **False.** IgG is associated with the secondary immune response.
   C. **True.**
   D. **False.** Serum IgG normally is about 70% IgG$_1$.
   E. **True.**

Suggested Reading
Hoffbrand and Lewis, Chapter 8, Blood group serology.

A4.16 A. **True.**
   B. **False.** The predominant cell is a promyelocyte.
   C. **False.** Sudan black staining is strongly positive.
   D. **False.** TdT staining is uniformly negative in M3.
   E. **True.** This is caused by release of a thromboplastin-like substance from the promyelocyte granules.

Suggested Reading
Hall and Malia, Chapter 13, The proliferative disorders.

Q4.17 The following differentiation antigens are markers of B lymphocytes:

A. CD22.
B. CD2.
C. CD33.
D. CD14.
E. CDw41.

Q4.18 The following statements relate to platelet prostaglandin metabolism:

A. arachidonic acid is converted to the prostaglandin PGG_2 by the enzyme cyclo-oxygenase.
B. prostaglandin H_2 is converted to thromboxane A_2 by the enzyme thromboxane synthetase.
C. thromboxane A_2 is a potent inhibitor of platelet aggregation.
D. cyclo-oxygenase is reversibly inhibited by acetylsalicylic acid (aspirin).
E. thromboxane A_2 is rapidly degraded to form prostacyclin PGI_2.

Q4.19 Bruton's agammaglobulinaemia

A. is inherited as an autosomal recessive condition.
B. is characterised by absolute lymphopenia.
C. is caused by failure of thymic development *in utero*.
D. is significantly associated with an increased incidence of auto-immune disease.
E. is characterised by deficiency of the enzyme adenine deaminase (ADA).

Q4.20 The following cytogenetic abnormalities are significantly associated with the myelodysplastic syndromes (MDS):

A. trisomy 8.
B. the translocation t(8;21).
C. monosomy 7.
D. the translocation t(15;17).
E. the deletion 5q-.

A4.17 A. **True.**
B. **False.** This is the sheep red cell receptor of T lymphocytes.
C. **False.** This is a marker of early myeloid precursors.
D. **False.** This is present on monocytes, macrophages and dendritic reticulum cells.
E. **False.** This is platelet glycoprotein IIb/IIIa.

Suggested Reading
Hall and Malia, Chapter 13, The proliferative disorders.

A4.18 A. **True.**
B. **True.**
C. **False.** TXA_2 is a potent promoter of platelet aggregation.
D. **False.** Aspirin irreversibly acetylates cyclo-oxygenase.
E. **False.** PGI_2 is a product of vascular endothelial prostaglandin metabolism. TXA_2 is degraded to TXB_2.

Suggested Reading
Hoffbrand and Lewis, Chapter 21, Normal haemostasis.

A4.19 A. **False.** This is inherited as an X-linked disorder.
B. **False.** Lymphopenia is an unusual finding.
C. **False.** This is DiGeorge syndrome.
D. **True.**
E. **False.** Deficiency of this enzyme leads to severe combined immunodeficiency (SCID).

Suggested Reading
Hoffbrand and Lewis, Chapter 12, Normal lymphocytes and their benign disorders.

A4.20 A. **True.**
B. **False.** This translocation is seen most commonly in M2. It is rare in MDS.
C. **True.**
D. **False.** This translocation appears to be specific for M3.
E. **True.**

Suggested Reading
Hoffbrand and Lewis, Chapter 17, The myelodysplastic syndromes.

Multiple Choice Test Five

Q5.1 Stainable iron deposits in the bone marrow characteristically are increased in the following conditions:

A. haemochromatosis.
B. chronic intravascular haemolysis.
C. transfusion-induced haemosiderosis.
D. haemolytic disease of the newborn (HDN).
E. primary acquired sideroblastic anaemia.

Q5.2 The following results are consistent with a diagnosis of severe haemophilia A:

A. a markedly prolonged APTT.
B. factor VIII_c assay of less than 1%.
C. a ristocetin cofactor assay (ricof) of 5%.
D. a markedly prolonged prothrombin time.
E. absence of platelet aggregation response to ADP *in vitro*.

Q5.3 The following blood film and bone marrow smear appearances are characteristic of severe megaloblastic anaemia:

A. uniform, round macrocytosis on the blood film.
B. giant metamyelocytes in the bone marrow smear.
C. a left shift in the neutrophils on the blood film.
D. bone marrow hyperplasia with signs of ineffective erythropoiesis.
E. leucopenia and thrombocytopenia on the blood film.

Q5.4 The following coagulation reactions require the presence of calcium ions:

A. stabilisation of fibrin by factor XIII.
B. the conversion of fibrinogen to fibrin monomer.
C. the formation of the prothrombinase complex.
D. contact activation of factor XII.
E. activation of factor VII in the presence of tissue factor.

A5.1   A. **True.**
        B. **True.**
        C. **True.**
        D. **True.**
        E. **True.**

Suggested Reading
Eastham, Chapter 3, Anaemia.

A5.2   A. **True.**   The APTT is a test of the extrinsic pathway.
        B. **True.**   This is essential for such a diagnosis.
        C. **False.** This is suggestive of von Willebrand's disease.
        D. **False.** The PT is most sensitive to deficiencies of factors II, VII, IX and X.
        E. **False.** Platelet aggregation is normal.

Suggested Reading
Hall and Malia, Chapter 16, Haemorrhagic disorders.

A5.3   A. **False.** The blood picture shows ovalomacrocytosis with gross anisocytosis.
        B. **True.**   These abnormal cells die in the bone marrow.
        C. **False.** The neutrophils typically show a right shift.
        D. **True.**
        E. **True.**

Suggested Reading
Hall and Malia, Chapter 10, Macrocytosis and the megaloblastic anaemias.

A5.4   A. **True.**
        B. **False.**
        C. **True.**
        D. **False.**
        E. **True.**

Suggested Reading
Hall and Malia, Chapter 2, Physiology of the blood.

Q5.5 **The following are neutrophil inclusion bodies:**

A. Russell bodies.
B. Howell-Jolly bodies.
C. Pappenheimer bodies.
D. Döhle bodies.
E. Heinz bodies.

Q5.6 **The following statements relate to the viscosity of normal plasma:**

A. the major determinant of plasma viscosity is the fibrinogen level.
B. the normal range of plasma viscosity at 25°C is 1.50-1.72 cP.
C. viscosity is defined as the ratio between shear stress and shear rate.
D. plasma behaves as a Newtonian fluid.
E. the plasma viscosity of neonates is normally lower than that of adults.

Q5.7 **The following statements relate to haemopoiesis in a 12-week-old foetus:**

A. the yolk sac is a major site of haemopoiesis.
B. the red cells have an MCV of about 90 fl.
C. red cell precursors are demonstrable in the bone marrow.
D. haemoglobin A is the major haemoglobin synthesised.
E. α globin chain production has begun to replace ζ globin chain production.

A5.5 A. **False.** These are seen in the plasma cells in myeloma.
B. **False.** These are red cell nuclear remnants.
C. **False.** These are iron-containing red cell inclusions.
D. **True.** These pale blue inclusions are seen in May-Hegglin anomaly and in scarlet fever.
E. **False.** These red cell inclusions consist of denatured globin.

Suggested Reading
Eastham, Chapter 4, Peripheral white cells.

A5.6 A. **True.** Fibrinogen is normally the most abundant plasma protein.
B. **True.**
C. **True.**
D. **True.** The viscosity of plasma is independent of the shear stress applied.
E. **True.** Neonates normally have lower levels of plasma immunoglobulins than adults.

Suggested Reading
Hall and Malia, Chapter 7, Erythrocyte sedimentation rate, plasma viscosity and blood rheology.

A5.7 A. **False.** The yolk sac ceases haemopoiesis at about 10 weeks gestation.
B. **False.** Erythropoiesis is macronormoblastic. The MCV is about 180 fl.
C. **True.**
D. **False.** Haemoglobin F is the major form produced.
E. **True.** α globin is demonstrable at 5 weeks gestation.

Suggested Reading
Hall and Malia, Chapter 2, Physiology of the blood.

Q5.8 The following are established causes of aplastic anaemia:

A. Epstein Barr virus.
B. chloramphenicol therapy.
C. exposure to ionising radiation.
D. human T-lymphotropic virus I (HTLV-I).
E. prolonged exposure to benzene.

Q5.9 The following haemolytic states are hereditary primary red cell membrane abnormalities:

A. hereditary spherocytosis (HS).
B. paroxysmal cold haemoglobinuria (PCH).
C. hereditary acanthocytosis.
D. hereditary pyropoikilocytosis.
E. paroxysmal nocturnal haemoglobinuria (PNH).

Q5.10 The following physiological changes cause a "right shift" in the oxygen dissociation curve of haemoglobin A:

A. a fall in blood pH.
B. hypothermia.
C. an increased level of 2,3-diphosphoglycerate (2,3-DPG).
D. deficiency of the enzyme hexokinase.
E. hypoxia due to a sudden fall in atmospheric oxygen tension.

Q5.11 Hereditary sideroblastic anaemia is characterised by the following features:

A. autosomal recessive inheritance.
B. uniform macrocytosis on the blood film.
C. defective haem synthesis.
D. marked ineffective erythropoiesis.
E. up to 40% ring sideroblasts in the bone marrow.

A5.8 A. **False.** Epstein Barr virus is the causative agent of glandular fever, Burkitt's lymphoma and naso-pharyngeal carcinoma.

  B. **True.** Treatment with this antibiotic induces aplasia in a significant number of patients.

  C. **True.** Ionising radiation causes direct damage to bone marrow cells.

  D. **False.** HTLV-I is causally related to a variant of acute T lymphoblastic leukaemia (ATLL).

  E. **True.**

Suggested Reading
Hall and Malia, Chapter 12, Refractory anaemias.

A5.9 A. **True.** HS is caused by spectrin deficiency.

  B. **False.** PCH is an autoimmune haemolytic anaemia.

  C. **False.** Hereditary acanthocytosis is caused by plasma a-β-lipoproteinaemia.

  D. **True.** HPP is caused by a defect of spectrin assembly.

  E. **False.** This is an acquired defect.

Suggested Reading
Hall and Malia, Chapter 11, Haemolytic anaemias.

A5.10 A. **True.** This is the Bohr effect.

  B. **False.** A fall in blood temperature causes a left shift.

  C. **True.** 2,3-DPG fixes haemoglobin A in the low-affinity configuration.

  D. **False.** This causes a deficiency of 2,3-DPG.

  E. **True.**

Suggested Reading
Hall and Malia, Chapter 2, Physiology of the blood.

A5.11 A. **False.** HSA is inherited as an X-linked disorder.

  B. **False.** The typical blood picture is dimorphic with prominent microcytosis.

  C. **True.** Various defects of haem synthesis have been described in this disorder.

  D. **False.** This is typical of primary acquired sideroblastic anaemia.

  E. **True.**

Suggested Reading
Hall and Malia, Chapter 12, Refractory anaemias.

Q5.12 Vascular endothelial cells are known to synthesise the following substances:

A. thromboxane A_2.
B. von Willebrand Factor (vWF).
C. prostacyclin (PGI_2).
D. prothrombin (factor II).
E. plasminogen activator.

Q5.13 The following features are characteristic of the blasts of M5a acute leukaemia (poorly-differentiated subtype):

A. chloroacetate esterase staining negative.
B. inconspicuous or absent nucleoli.
C. scanty cytoplasm.
D. acid phosphatase staining negative.
E. a markedly raised serum lysozyme level.

Q5.14 The following parasites invade red cells:

A. *Babesia microti.*
B. *Wuchereria bancrofti.*
C. *Plasmodium ovale.*
D. *Trypanosoma cruzi.*
E. *Loa loa.*

Q5.15 The following features are characteristic of the myelodysplastic syndrome refractory anaemia with excess of blasts (RAEB):

A. Auer rods present in the bone marrow.
B. at least 5% blasts in the bone marrow smear.
C. hypocellular bone marrow.
D. at least 20% ring sideroblasts in the bone marrow.
E. less than 5% blasts in the peripheral blood.

A5.12 A. **False.** This is a product of platelet metabolism.
        B. **True.**
        C. **True.**
        D. **False.** This is synthesised by hepatocytes.
        E. **True.**

Suggested Reading
Hoffbrand and Lewis, Chapter 21, Normal haemostasis.

A5.13 A. **True.** This is a granulocyte marker.
        B. **False.** The blasts typically have 1-3 large, vesicular nucleoli.
        C. **False.** The cytoplasm typically is plentiful.
        D. **False.** Acid phosphatase staining is strongly positive.
        E. **False.** Lysozyme is expressed by more mature monocyte precursors.

Suggested Reading
Hall and Malia, Chapter 13, The proliferative disorders.

A5.14 A. **True.**
        B. **False.**
        C. **True.**
        D. **False.**
        E. **False.**

Suggested Reading
Hall and Malia, Chapter 14, Haematology of infections.

A5.15 A. **False.** The presence of Auer rods is characteristic of RAEB-t.
        B. **True.**
        C. **False.** The bone marrow typically is normo- or hypercellular.
        D. **False.** This is characteristic of RAEB-t.
        E. **True.**

Suggested Reading
Hoffbrand and Lewis, Chapter 17, The myelodysplastic syndromes.

Q5.16 **The following conditions characteristically lead to increased circulating levels of methaemoglobin:**

A. NADH-linked methaemoglobin reductase I deficiency.
B. the administration of 400 mg of ascorbic acid (vitamin C) daily.
C. severe chronic intravascular haemolysis.
D. the presence of haemoglobin Boston.
E. treatment with oxidising drugs such as sulphonamides in a neonate.

Q5.17 **The following statements relate to the Embden-Meyerhof pathway of the normal mature red cell:**

A. the conversion of glucose to glucose-6-phosphate (G-6-P) is catalysed by the enzyme hexokinase.
B. there is a net loss of energy in the conversion of glucose to lactate.
C. pyruvate kinase (PK) catalyses the conversion of 1,3-diphosphoglycerate (1,3-DPG) to 3-phosphoglycerate (3-PG).
D. the NADH formed via this pathway helps to maintain the ferrous (Fe^{2+}) ion in haem in its reduced state.
E. the Rappaport-Luebering shunt results in the formation of 2,3-diphosphoglycerate (2,3-DPG).

Q5.18 **The following statements relate to the structure of normal metaphase chromosomes in man:**

A. the two sister chromatids of each chromosome meet at the telomere.
B. there are nine groups of morphologically similar chromosomes, designated as groups A-I.
C. the long arms of the chromosome are designated the p arms.
D. telocentric chromosomes have a central centromere.
E. the largest of the autosomes is chromosome 7.

A5.16 A. **True.** This enzyme catalyses the reduction of methaemoglobin.
  B. **False.** Vitamin C is a reducing agent which is used in the treatment of methaemoglobinaemia.
  C. **True.**
  D. **True.** Hb Boston is one of the HbMs.
  E. **True.** Neonates have reduced levels of NADH-linked methaemoglobin reductase.

Suggested Reading
Hall and Malia, Chapter 11, Haemolytic anaemias.

A5.17 A. **True.**
  B. **False.** There is a net gain of 2 mol of ATP per mol of glucose metabolised.
  C. **False.** PK catalyses the conversion of phosphoenolpyruvate to pyruvate.
  D. **True.** NADH acts as a cofactor for the enzyme methaemoglobin reductase.
  E. **True.**

Suggested Reading
Hall and Malia, Chapter 2, Physiology of the blood.

A5.18 A. **False.** The chromatids meet at the centromere.
  B. **False.** There are seven groups (A-G).
  C. **False.** The long arms are designated q.
  D. **False.** Chromosomes with a central centromere are termed metacentric. Telocentric chromosomes have their centromere at one end.
  E. **False.** Chromosome 1 is the largest autosome.

Suggested Reading
Hoffbrand and Lewis, Chapter 13, Cytogenetics and leukaemogenesis.

Q5.19   DiGeorge syndrome

A. is inherited as an autosomal recessive condition.
B. is due to thymic aplasia.
C. is caused by deficiency of the enzyme purine nucleoside phosphorylase.
D. typically is associated with severe hypogammaglobulinaemia.
E. is characterised by recurrent fungal, viral and mycobacterial infection.

Q5.20   The following statements relate to molecular defects in the α thalassaemia syndromes:

A. the majority of α thalassaemias result from point mutations within the α gene complex.
B. the ζ gene is not deleted in most α^o homozygotes.
C. most non-deletion forms of α thalassaemia affect the $\alpha 1$ gene.
D. haemoglobin Constant Spring results from a point mutation of the $\alpha 2$ gene "stop" codon.
E. haemoglobin Quong Sze is an α chain variant which results in post-translational instability and so an α thalassaemia phenotype.

A5.19 A. **False.** DiGeorge syndrome is not inherited.
   B. **True.** It is caused by failure of development of the 3rd and 4th pharyngeal pouches *in utero*.
   C. **False.**
   D. **False.** Immunoglobulin levels typically are normal in this condition.
   E. **True.** Lack of T cells renders the host susceptible to these organisms.

Suggested Reading
Hoffbrand and Lewis, Chapter 12, Normal lymphocytes and their benign disorders.

A5.20 A. **False.** Most α thalassaemias result from deletions.
   B. **True.** This allows synthesis of Hb Portland ($\zeta_2\gamma_2$) *in utero*.
   C. **False.** Most non-deletion α thalassaemias affect the α2 gene.
   D. **True.** This results in an α globin chain which is 31 amino acids longer than normal.
   E. **True.**

Suggested Reading
Hall and Malia, Chapter 9, Microcytic anaemias.

Multiple Choice Test Six

Q6.1   A "left shift" of the neutrophils is a recognised
feature of

A. untreated chronic myeloid leukaemia.
B. severe megaloblastic anaemia due to folate deficiency.
C. acute bacterial infection.
D. Pelger-Huët phenomenon.
E. chronic granulomatous disease (CGD).

Q6.2   The following statements relate to the structure
of haemoglobin A:

A. it has the composition $\alpha_2\delta_2$.
B. it accounts for up to 80% of the total haemoglobin in a
normal adult.
C. each molecule contains one haem group.
D. α globin contains 141 amino acid residues.
E. each HbA molecule is capable of binding one molecule
of oxygen.

Q6.3   The following statements relate to blood products:

A. platelet concentrates are best stored at 4°C.
B. cryoprecipitate is rich in coagulation factor IX.
C. human plasma protein fraction (HPPF) is rich in
coagulation factors.
D. fresh frozen plasma (FFP) must be thawed at 56°C
before use.
E. blood for exchange transfusion of a neonate must be at
least 6 days old.

Q6.4   The following statements relate to the iron-binding
protein transferrin:

A. it has a molecular weight of 76,000-80,000 daltons.
B. it binds four atoms of iron per molecule of transferrin.
C. the normal adult total iron binding capacity (TIBC)
is 45-72 μmol/l.
D. plasma transferrin is normally 90-95% saturated with
iron in a healthy adult.
E. congenital atransferrinaemia presents as a severe
hypochromic anaemia in infancy.

59

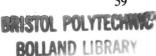

A6.1 A. **True.**

        B. **False.**   Megaloblastic anaemia is associated with neutrophil hypersegmentation (ie a right shift).

        C. **True.**

        D. **True.**   This inherited condition is associated with hyposegmentation.

        E. **False.**   CGD neutrophils are morphologically normal.

Suggested Reading

Hall and Malia, Chapter 2, Physiology of the blood.

A6.2 A. **False.**   It has the composition $\alpha_2\beta_2$.

        B. **False.**   It accounts for about 96% of the total.

        C. **False.**   Each globin chain is associated with one haem group ie four in total.

        D. **True.**

        E. **False.**   Each molecule can bind up to four O_2 molecules.

Suggested Reading

Hall and Malia, Chapter 2, Physiology of the blood.

A6.3 A. **False.**   Post-transfusion survival is poor if the platelets are stored at 4°C. They should be stored at room temperature.

        B. **False.**   Cryoprecipitate contains mainly factors VIII_c, vWF, fibrinogen and some XIII.

        C. **False.**   HPPF contains no coagulation factors.

        D. **False.**   Incubation at 56°C denatures coagulation factors.

        E. **False.**   Blood for exchange transfusion should be as fresh as possible to minimise the risk of hyperkalaemia.

Suggested Reading

Hoffbrand and Lewis, Chapter 10, Clinical blood transfusion.

A6.4 A. **True.**

        B. **False.**   Transferrin has two non-identical binding sites.

        C. **True.**

        D. **False.**   Transferrin is normally about 30-35% saturated with iron.

        E. **True.**

Suggested Reading

Hoffbrand and Lewis, Chapter 2, Iron.

Q6.5 Aluminium hydroxide adsorbs the following coagulation factors from plasma:

A. factor I (fibrinogen).
B. factor II (prothrombin).
C. factor XII.
D. factor VII.
E. factor VIII_c.

Q6.6 The following substances are suitable for routine use as anticoagulants in coagulation studies:

A. lithium heparin.
B. trisodium citrate.
C. dipotassium EDTA.
D. HEPES buffer.
E. a mixture of potassium and ammonium oxalates.

Q6.7 The following conditions characteristically result in increased red cell deformability *in vivo*:

A. hereditary spherocytosis (HS).
B. the presence of large numbers of Heinz bodies.
C. sickle cell disease.
D. a diet rich in fish oils over a prolonged period.
E. severe hypothermia.

Q6.8 The following conditions are characterised by a low level of factor VIII_c:

A. von Willebrand's disease:
B. alcoholic liver disease.
C. haemophilia A.
D. pseudo von Willebrand's disease.
E. Bernard-Soulier syndrome.

A6.5 A. **False.** Al(OH)$_3$ adsorbs factors II, VII, IX and X.
       B. **True.**
       C. **False.**
       D. **True.**
       E. **False.**

Suggested Reading
Hall and Malia, Chapter 15, Basic principles of
haemostatic testing.

A6.6 A. **False.** Heparin prolongs coagulation times, even after
                  recalcification.
       B. **True.** This is the anticoagulant of choice for
                  routine work.
       C. **False.** VIII$_c$ is highly unstable in EDTA.
       D. **False.** HEPES is sometimes added to citrate to stabilise
                  pH but has no anticoagulant properties of its own.
       E. **False.** V is highly unstable in oxalate.

Suggested Reading
Hall and Malia, Chapter 15, Basic principles of
haemostatic testing.

A6.7 A. **False.** Spherocytes are more rigid than biconcave discs.
       B. **False.** Red cell inclusions decrease deformability.
       C. **False.** Sickle cells are rigid and inflexible.
       D. **True.** Fish oil is taken up by the red cell membrane
                  and increases its deformability.
       E. **False.** Red cells are less deformable at low temperature.

Suggested Reading
Eastham, Chapter 2, Red blood cells.

A6.8 A. **True.** VIII$_c$ is destroyed in the circulation because
                  of the deficiency of its carrier protein, vWF.
       B. **False.** VIII$_c$ levels typically are normal or raised in
                  alcoholic liver disease.
       C. **True.**
       D. **True.** see A.
       E. **False.** This is due to deficiency of platelet
                  glycoprotein Ib.

Suggested Reading
Hall and Malia, Chapter 16, Haemorrhagic disorders.

Q6.9 The following features are consistent with a diagnosis of myelofibrosis:

A. massive splenomegaly.
B. marked thrombocytosis.
C. leucoerythroblastic blood picture.
D. decreased plasma volume.
E. extramedullary haemopoiesis.

Q6.10 The following substances contain iron:

A. myoglobin.
B. hydroxycobalamin.
C. catalase.
D. cyclo-oxygenase.
E. cytochrome b_2.

Q6.11 The following statements relate to the heterophil antibodies in human serum in health and disease:

A. the Forsmann antibody is adsorbed by ox red cell stroma.
B. the heterophil antibody of serum sickness is adsorbed by guinea-pig kidney suspension.
C. the heterophil antibody of glandular fever is adsorbed by guinea-pig kidney suspension.
D. horse red cells are agglutinated by the heterophil antibody of glandular fever.
E. mouse red cells are agglutinated by Forsmann antibody.

Q6.12 The following laboratory results are consistent with a diagnosis of heterozygous α^+ thalassaemia ($\alpha\alpha/\alpha$-):

A. 1% haemoglobin Barts in the cord blood.
B. raised levels of haemoglobins A_2 and F in an adult.
C. haemoglobin H inclusions demonstrable in most red cells.
D. a moderate microcytic, hypochromic anaemia.
E. 5% haemoglobin Portland in an adult.

63

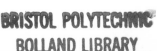

A6.9   A. **True.**   Splenomegaly reflects extramedullary
                          haemopoiesis.
         B. **True.**   Extreme thrombocytosis with bizarre morphology
                          is often present at diagnosis.
         C. **True.**   This is a characteristic finding.
         D. **False.**   Plasma volume typically is raised.
         E. **True.**

Suggested Reading
   Hoffbrand and Lewis, Chapter 20, Non-leukaemic
   myeloproliferative disorders.

A6.10   A. **True.**   Myoglobin contains haem.
         B. **False.**   Hydroxycobalamin contains cobalt.
         C. **True.**   Catalase contains haem.
         D. **True.**   Cyclo-oxygenase contains haem.
         E. **True.**   Cytochrome b_2 contains haem.

Suggested Reading
   Eastham, Chapter 3, Anaemia.

A6.11   A. **False.**
         B. **True.**
         C. **False.**
         D. **True.**
         E. **True.**

Suggested Reading
   Hall and Malia, Chapter 14, Haematology of infections.

A6.12   A. **True.**
         B. **False.**   This is suggestive of β thalassaemia.
         C. **False.**   This is typical of HbH disease (α-/--).
         D. **False.**   The absolute values typically are normal
                          or only minimally decreased.
         E. **False.**   Hb Portland is an embryonic haemoglobin.

Suggested Reading
   Hall and Malia, Chapter 9, Microcytic anaemias.

Q6.13 The following peripheral blood film appearances are consistent with a diagnosis of *Plasmodium falciparum* malaria:

A. Schüffner's dots.
B. crescent-shaped gametocytes.
C. Maurer's dots.
D. double chromatin dots in the trophozoites.
E. the red cells containing schizonts are greatly enlarged.

Q6.14 Whole blood viscosity

A. is higher in capillaries than arteries.
B. is higher at low shear rates.
C. is raised in hypofibrinogenaemia.
D. is increased in homozygous haemoglobin C disease.
E. typically is raised post-splenectomy.

Q6.15 The following unstable haemoglobins result from substitution of haem contact amino acids:

A. haemoglobin Köln (β 98 (FG5) val–>meth).
B. haemoglobin Bristol (β 67 (E11) val–>asp).
C. haemoglobin Sabine (β 19 (F7) leu–>pro).
D. haemoglobin Hammersmith (β 42 (CD1) phe–>ser).
E. haemoglobin Philly (β 35 (E1) tyr–>phen).

Q6.16 Serum folate levels characteristically are reduced in the following conditions, assuming absence of prophylaxis:

A. chronic haemolysis of moderate severity.
B. in patients undergoing peritoneal dialysis.
C. in babies fed exclusively on goat's milk.
D. coeliac disease.
E. in long-term phenytoin (Epanutin) therapy.

A6.13   A. **False.**   Schüffner's dots are seen in *P. vivax* or
                           P. ovale malaria.
          B. **True.**   This is a characteristic finding.
          C. **True.**
          D. **True.**   These are most common in *P. falciparum* malaria.
          E. **False.**   Infected red cells are of normal size.

Suggested Reading
     Hall and Malia, Chapter 14, Haematology of infections.

A6.14   A. **True.**
          B. **True.**   Whole blood is thixotropic.
          C. **False.**   Plasma viscosity (and hence WBV) is decreased
                           in hypofibrinogenaemia.
          D. **True.**   Target cells are poorly deformable.
          E. **True.**   Red cell inclusions decrease deformability.

Suggested Reading
     Hall and Malia, Chapter 7, Erythrocyte sedimentation rate,
     plasma viscosity and blood rheology.

A6.15   A. **True.**
          B. **False.**   This molecule is unstable due to substitution
                           of a non-polar by a polar amino acid with
                           resultant distortion of the haem pocket.
          C. **False.**   This molecule is unstable due to the
                           substitution of proline in a helical portion.
          D. **True.**
          E. **False.**   This molecule results from a substitution at
                           the $\alpha_1\beta_1$ contact.

Suggested Reading
     Hall and Malia, Chapter 11, Haemolytic anaemias.

A6.16   A. **True.**   Deficiency results from increased utilisation.
          B. **True.**   Folate is lost in the dialysate.
          C. **True.**   Goat's milk is a poor source of folate.
          D. **True.**   This disorder is characterised by malabsorption
                           of folate.
          E. **True.**   Phenytoin interferes with intestinal
                           absorption of folate.

Suggested Reading
     Hoffbrand and Lewis, Chapter 3, Megaloblastic anaemia.

Q6.17   Epoprostenol (PGI$_2$)

A. is synthesised by platelets from arachidonic acid.
B. is a powerful platelet aggregating agent.
C. synthesis is inhibited by circulating "lupus" anticoagulant.
D. acts as a vasodilator.
E. acts by increasing platelet cAMP levels.

**Q6.18   The following statements relate to the sub-types
of von Willebrand's disease:**

A. type IIA is characterised by absence of low molecular
weight multimers of vWF.
B. type IIB is characterised by increased platelet aggregation
response to ristocetin.
C. the electrophoretic mobility of vWF is increased in type I.
D. all multimeric forms of vWF are present in type IIC.
E. VIII$_c$ synthesis is normal in type III.

**Q6.19   The following substances are recognised chemotactic
factors for neutrophils in man:**

A. the Complement component C3$_a$.
B. phytohaemagglutinin.
C. the Complement component C5$_a$.
D. leukotriene B.
E. interleukin-3 (IL-3).

Q6.20   Interleukin-2 (IL-2)

A. is synthesised by macrophages.
B. is only produced during S phase of the cell cycle.
C. acts mainly on unprimed lymphocytes.
D. has a molecular weight of 15,000 daltons.
E. is used to stimulate production of T-lymphocytes
in *in vitro* culture.

A6.17 A. **False.** PGI_2 is a product of vascular endothelium.
       B. **False.** It is a powerful inhibitor of platelet aggregation.
       C. **True.** Deficiency of PGI_2 may contribute to the thrombotic tendency seen with lupus anticoagulant.
       D. **True.**
       E. **True.**

Suggested Reading
Hoffbrand and Lewis, Chapter 21, Normal haemostasis.

A6.18 A. **False.** Absence of large and intermediate multimers is typical.
       B. **True.**
       C. **False.** Electrophoretic mobility is normal in type I.
       D. **False.** Absence of large multimers and an abnormal multimeric pattern is typical.
       E. **True.** VIII_c synthesis is normal in all sub-types.

Suggested Reading
Hoffbrand and Lewis, Chapter 23, Inherited bleeding disorders.

A6.19 A. **True.**
       B. **False.** PHA is a lymphocyte mitogenic factor.
       C. **True.**
       D. **True.**
       E. **False.** IL-3 is a haemopoietic growth factor. Murine neutrophils carry an IL-3 receptor but human neutrophils do not.

Suggested Reading
Roitt, Brostoff and Male, Chapter 1, Adaptive and innate immunity.

A6.20 A. **False.** IL-2 is generated by T helper cells.
       B. **False.** It can be generated by non-dividing cells.
       C. **False.** It has no effect on unprimed lymphocytes.
       D. **False.** It has a molecular weight of about 30,000 daltons.
       E. **True.** Macrophages must also be present.

Suggested Reading
Roitt, Brostoff and Male, Chapter 8, Cell cooperation in the immune response.

Multiple Choice Test Seven

Q7.1 The following conditions are inherited as X-linked disorders:

A. haemophilia A (VIII$_c$ deficiency).
B. hereditary sideroblastic anaemia.
C. von Willebrand's disease (type I).
D. chronic granulomatous disease of childhood (CGD).
E. hereditary haemorrhagic telangiectasia (HHT).

Q7.2 The following are red cell inclusion bodies:

A. Howell-Jolly bodies.
B. Döhle bodies.
C. Pappenheimer bodies.
D. Russell bodies.
E. Maurer's dots.

Q7.3 A normal 38-week-old foetus is synthesising the following haemoglobins or haemoglobin precursors:

A. haemoglobin Gower I.
B. δ globin chains.
C. ε globin chains.
D. haemoglobin Barts.
E. ζ globin chains.

Q7.4 Intestinal absorption of dietary non-haem iron is facilitated by:

A. high doses of vitamin C with meals.
B. pancreatic secretions.
C. achlorhydria.
D. decreased duodenal pH.
E. high concentrations of phosphate in the food.

A7.1 A. **True.**
  B. **True.** A rare autosomal form also exists.
  C. **False.** VWD is inherited as an autosomal dominant condition.
  D. **True.** A rare autosomal recessive form also exists.
  E. **False.** HHT is an autosomal dominant condition.

Suggested Reading
  Hoffbrand and Lewis, Chapter 23, Inherited bleeding disorders.
  Hoffbrand and Lewis, Chapter 11, Granulocytes, monocytes and their benign disorders.

A7.2 A. **True.**
  B. **False.** These inclusion bodies are seen in the neutrophils in May-Hegglin anomaly.
  C. **True.**
  D. **False.** These are plasma cell inclusions.
  E. **True.** These are seen in *P. falciparum* malaria.

Suggested Reading
  Eastham, Chapter 2, Red blood cells.

A7.3 A. **False.** Hb Gower I is synthesised up to 10/40.
  B. **True.**
  C. **False.** ε chains are synthesised up to 10/40.
  D. **False.** Hb Barts is only seen in α thalassaemia.
  E. **False.** ζ chains are synthesised up to 10/40.

Suggested Reading
  Hall and Malia, Chapter 1, Haemopoiesis.

A7.4 A. **True.** Vitamin C is a reducing agent.
  B. **False.** Pancreatic secretions are alkaline.
  C. **False.**
  D. **True.** Fe^{3+} is converted to Fe^{2+} at acid pH.
  E. **False.** Phosphate inhibits iron absorption.

Suggested Reading
  Hoffbrand and Lewis, Chapter 2, Iron.

Q7.5   Siderocytes in the peripheral blood are a recognised
feature of the following conditions:

A. acute lead poisoning.
B. severe iron deficiency.
C. pernicious anaemia (PA).
D. newborn, premature infants.
E. homozygous β^+ thalassaemia.

Q7.6   The following laboratory results are consistent with a
diagnosis of pernicious anaemia (PA):

A. a serum vitamin B_{12} level of 850 ng/l.
B. microcytosis with target cells on the blood film.
C. severe bone marrow hypoplasia.
D. auto-antibodies directed against gastric parietal cells
   demonstrable in the serum.
E. excretion of more than 50% of the test dose in a Schilling
   test without added intrinsic factor.

Q7.7   Neutrophil primary granules contain the following
substances:

A. acid phosphatase.
B. myeloperoxidase.
C. β-glucuronidase.
D. lysozyme.
E. lactoferrin.

Q7.8   The following conditions typically result in an increased
total red cell volume (TRCV):

A. persistent, severe diarrhoea and vomiting.
B. normal, uncomplicated pregnancy.
C. polycythaemia rubra vera (PRV).
D. severe, chronic pulmonary disease.
E. Gaisbock's syndrome.

A7.5   A. **True.**   Haem synthesis is disrupted in lead poisoning.

         B. **False.**   Siderotic granules contain iron and so are not seen in iron deficiency.

         C. **True.**

         D. **True.**   Siderocytes are normally present during the first few days of life.

         E. **True.**

Suggested Reading

     Eastham, Chapter 2, Red blood cells.

A7.6   A. **False.**   The normal range for serum B_{12} is 170-850 ng/l.

         B. **False.**   PA typically is a macrocytic anaemia.

         C. **False.**   The marrow typically is hyperplastic with ineffective erythropoiesis..

         D. **True.**   Parietal cell antibodies are demonstrable in 90% of cases.

         E. **False.**   Less than 5% of the test dose is excreted in in the absence of intrinsic factor in PA.

Suggested Reading

     Hall and Malia, Chapter 10, Macrocytosis and the megaloblastic anaemias.

A7.7   A. **True.**

         B. **True.**

         C. **True.**

         D. **False.**   Lysozyme is a secondary granule constituent.

         E. **False.**   Lactoferrin is a secondary granule constituent.

Suggested Reading

     Hoffbrand and Lewis, Chapter 11, Granulocytes, monocytes and their benign disorders.

A7.8   A. **False.**   This leads to a reduction in plasma volume due to dehydration.

         B. **True.**   Red cell mass typically increases by up to 40% by 32 weeks gestation.

         C. **True.**   A raised TRCV is characteristic of PRV.

         D. **True.**   The increased red cell mass in this condition is secondary to hypoxia.

         E. **False.**   The red cell mass is normal in this condition.

Suggested Reading

     Hoffbrand and Lewis, Chapter 20, Non-leukaemic myeloproliferative disorders.

Q7.9 The following substances are known to potentiate the anticoagulant activity of warfarin:

A. alcohol.
B. oral contraceptives.
C. sulphonamides.
D. anabolic steroids.
E. barbiturates.

Q7.10 The following laboratory results are characteristic of homozygous β° thalassaemia:

A. marked ineffective erythropoiesis.
B. haemoglobin A levels of 25-30%.
C. severe microcytic, hypochromic anaemia.
D. at least 25% ringed sideroblasts in the bone marrow.
E. haemoglobin F levels of 30-40% in an adult.

Q7.11 The following statements relate to coagulation factor VII:

A. the activated form (VII_a) is a two-chain molecule linked by disulphide bridges.
B. vitamin K catalyses the carboxylation of lysine residues in the molecule, rendering it capable of binding calcium ions.
C. it is absent from serum.
D. it has the shortest *in vivo* half life of all the coagulation factors.
E. it has the electrophoretic mobility of an α globulin.

Q7.12 The following statements relate to inherited disorders of platelet function:

A. Bernard-Soulier syndrome is inherited as an autosomal dominant character.
B. Glanzmann's thrombasthenia is caused by a deficiency of platelet glycoproteins IIb/IIIa.
C. Grey platelet syndrome is characterised by a deficiency of platelet α granules.
D. ristocetin-induced platelet aggregation *in vitro* characteristically is reduced in Bernard-Soulier syndrome.
E. Glanzmann's thrombasthenia is characterised by severe thrombocytopenia.

73

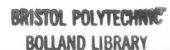

A7.9   A. **True.**   Alcohol increases the plasma half-life of warfarin
       B. **False.**   Oral contraceptives cause an increased synthesis of coagulation factors.
       C. **True.**   Sulphonamides decrease the binding of warfarin to serum albumin.
       D. **True.**   Anabolic steroids induce increased synthesis of coagulation factors.
       E. **False.**   Barbiturates enhance the rate of hepatic degradation of warfarin.

Suggested Reading
Hoffbrand and Lewis, Chapter 25, Thrombosis and antithrombotic therapy.

A7.10   A. **True.**
       B. **False.**   HbA is absent.
       C. **True.**
       D. **False.**   Ringed sideroblasts are not a feature of this disorder.
       E. **False.**   The HbF level is about 98%.

Suggested Reading
Hall and Malia, Chapter 9, Microcytic anaemias.

A7.11   A. **False.** VII_a is a single chain glycoprotein.
       B. **False.**   Vitamin K catalyses the carboxylation of glutamyl residues.
       C. **False.**
       D. **True.**
       E. **False.**   VII migrates with the β globulins on electrophoresis.

Suggested Reading
Hoffbrand and Lewis, Chapter 21, Normal haemostasis.

A7.12   A. **False.**   BSS is inherited as an autosomal recessive condition.
       B. **True.**
       C. **True.**
       D. **True.**
       E. **False.**   The platelet count typically is normal in Glanzmann's thrombasthenia.

Suggested Reading
Hoffbrand and Lewis, Chapter 22, Platelet disorders.

Q7.13 The following micro-organisms are recognised as suitable for use in the assay of the stated substance:

A. *Euglena gracilis* in the assay of vitamin B_{12}.
B. *Listeria monocytogenes* in the assay of pteroyl glutamic acid (PGA).
C. *Lactobacillus leichmannii* in the assay of tetrahydrofolate.
D. *Pediococcus cerevisiae* in the assay of vitamin B_{12}.
E. *Lactobacillus casei* in the assay of serum and red cell folate.

Q7.14 The following laboratory results are characteristic of the blast cells of T-acute lymphoblastic leukaemia (T-ALL):

A. cytoplasmic IgM (CIg) demonstrable by immunofluorescence.
B. staining for terminal deoxynucleotidyl transferase (TdT) negative.
C. staining for CD10 positive.
D. surface immunoglobulin (SIg) demonstrable by immunofluorescence.
E. staining for Ia antigen positive.

Q7.15 Circulating levels of Antithrombin III (ATIII) typically are decreased in the following circumstances:

A. premature neonates.
B. during effective intravenous heparin therapy.
C. during effective L-asparaginase therapy.
D. decompensated disseminated intravascular coagulation (DIC).
E. during effective warfarin therapy.

Q7.16 The following statements relate to red cell membrane lipids:

A. the most abundant membrane lipid is unesterified cholesterol.
B. sphingomyelin is restricted to the inner (cytosol) layer of the membrane.
C. mature red cells actively synthesise lipid for membrane repair.
D. membrane cholesterol exchanges freely with its plasma counterpart.
E. phosphatidyl choline is located mainly in the outer (plasma) layer of the membrane.

A7.13   A. **True.**   *Euglena gracilis* is suitable for the assay of all physiological forms of vitamin B_{12}.

       B. **False.**   *Listeria monocytogenes* is not suitable for use in the assay of folate.

       C. **False.**   *Lactobacillus leichmannii* is used in the assay of vitamin B_{12}.

       D. **False.**   *Pediococcus cerevisiae* can be used in the assay of all tetrahydrofolates except 5-methyl THF.

       E. **True.**   *Lactobacillus casei* is the most suitable organism for the microbiological assay of folate.

Suggested Reading

Hall and Malia, Chapter 10, Macrocytosis and the megaloblastic anaemias.

A7.14   A. **False.**   This is a marker of pre-B ALL.

       B. **False.**

       C. **False.**   CD10 is the cALL antigen.

       D. **False.**

       E. **False.**

Suggested Reading

Hall and Malia, Chapter 13, The proliferative disorders.

A7.15   A. **True.**   ATII levels are about 30% in a 32-week gestation premature neonate.

       B. **True.**

       C. **True.**

       D. **True.**

       E. **False.**   ATIII levels typically are increased during warfarin therapy.

Suggested Reading

Hall and Malia, Chapter 17, Thrombosis.

A7.16   A. **True.**

       B. **False.**   It is mainly present in the plasma layer.

       C. **False.**   Mature red cells are incapable of lipid synthesis.

       D. **True.**

       E. **True.**

Suggested Reading

Hall and Malia, Chapter 2, Physiology of the blood.

Q7.17 The following cells are responsive to the action of erythropoietin:

A. CFU-GEMM.
B. BFU-E
C. the mature erythrocyte.
D. GM-CFU.
E. CFU-E.

Q7.18 The following chromosomal abnormalities are significantly associated with the stated disease:

A. t(9q+;22q-) with chronic myeloid leukaemia.
B. t(15q+,17q-) with acute promyelocytic leukaemia (M3).
C. monosomy 7 with chronic lymphocytic leukaemia.
D. t(8q-,14q+) with Burkitt's lymphoma.
E. trisomy 8 with chronic myeloid leukaemia.

Q7.19 Protein C activity characteristically is decreased in the following circumstances:

A. decompensated disseminated intravascular coagulation (DIC).
B. idiopathic thrombocytopenic purpura (ITP).
C. during effective warfarin therapy.
D. chronic liver disease.
E. in the third trimester of a normal pregnancy.

Q7.20 Arachidonic acid

A. is the most abundant unsaturated fatty acid in platelets.
B. is cleaved from platelet membrane phospholipids by the enzyme phospholipase A_2.
C. induces aggregation *in vitro* of aspirin-treated platelets.
D. is converted to prostacyclin (PGI_2) within platelets.
E. will induce aggregation *in vitro* in platelets from a case of Glanzmann's thrombasthenia.

A7.17 A. **False.** The earliest responsive precursor is the BFU-E.
       B. **True.**
       C. **False.**
       D. **False.** This cell can only differentiate into
                      granulocytes and macrophages.
       E. **True.**

Suggested Reading
Hoffbrand and Lewis, Chapter 1, Erythropoiesis.

A7.18 A. **True.**   This is the Philadelphia chromosome.
       B. **True.**   This is specific for M3.
       C. **False.** This is a common abnormality in the
                      myelodysplastic syndromes.
       D. **True.**
       E. **True.**   Trisomy 8 often develops as the disease
                      progresses.

Suggested Reading
Hoffbrand and Lewis, Chapter 13, Cytogenetics and
leukaemogenesis.

A7.19 A. True.
       B. False.
       C. True.   Protein C is vitamin K-dependent.
       D. True.   Protein C is synthesised in the liver.
       E. False.   There is no consistent change in pregnancy.

Suggested Reading
Hoffbrand and Lewis, Chapter 25, Thrombosis and
antithrombotic therapy.

A7.20 A. True.
       B. True.
       C. False. Arachidonic acid stimulates aggregation of
                  platelets via TXA_2 synthesis which is absent
                  from aspirin-treated platelets.
       D. True.   Prostacyclin is a product of prostaglandin
                  metabolism in vascular endothelial cells.
       E. False.

Suggested Reading
Hoffbrand and Lewis, Chapter 21, Normal haemostasis.

Multiple Choice Test Eight

Q8.1 Absolute leucopenia is a recognised feature of the following conditions:

A. paroxysmal nocturnal haemoglobinuria (PNH).
B. Wiskott-Aldrich syndrome.
C. chronic granulomatous disease (CGD).
D. Fanconi's anaemia.
E. Chediak-Higashi-Steinbrinck syndrome.

Q8.2 An absolute lymphocytosis is characteristic of the following conditions:

A. untreated acquired immune deficiency syndrome (AIDS).
B. *Salmonella* infection in an adult.
C. chronic lymphocytic leukaemia (CLL).
D. stage I Hodgkin's disease.
E. whooping cough (pertussis).

Q8.3 The following conditions characteristically display an increased myeloid:erythroid (M:E) ratio in the bone marrow:

A. Blackfan-Diamond syndrome.
B. untreated chronic myeloid leukaemia.
C. homozygous β^{o} thalassaemia.
D. anaemia of chronic renal failure.
E. drug-induced agranulocytosis.

Q8.4 Cryoprecipitate is rich in the following coagulation factors:

A. factor VII.
B. factor II (prothrombin).
C. VIII_{c}.
D. factor IX.
E. factor XI.

A8.1　A. **True.**
　　　B. **False.**
　　　C. **False.**　The white cell count typically is normal in CGD.
　　　D. **True.**　The white cell count may be normal at diagnosis but leucopenia generally develops.
　　　E. **True.**

Suggested Reading
　　Eastham, Chapter 4, Peripheral white blood cells.

A8.2　A. **False.**　Lymphopenia is more common.
　　　B. **False.**　Bacterial infections usually elicit a neutrophil leucocytosis.
　　　C. **True.**
　　　D. **False.**　The full blood count typically is normal at this stage of the disease.
　　　E. **True.**　Extreme lymphocytosis is common in pertussis.

Suggested Reading
　　Eastham, Chapter 4, Peripheral white blood cells.

A8.3　A. **True.**　This is pure red cell aplasia.
　　　B. **True.**　CML is characterised by an increased number of myeloid precursors in the bone marrow.
　　　C. **False.**　Erythroid hyperplasia with ineffective erythropoiesis is typical of this disorder.
　　　D. **True.**　CRF is accompanied by failure of erythropoietin production and erythroid hypoplasia.
　　　E. **False.**

Suggested Reading
　　Eastham, Chapter 5, Bone marrow.

A8.4　A. **False.**　Cryoprecipitate contains VIII_c, vWF, fibrinogen, fibronectin and some XIII.
　　　B. **False.**
　　　C. **True.**
　　　D. **False.**
　　　E. **False.**

Suggested Reading
　　Hoffbrand and Lewis, Chapter 10, Clinical blood transfusion.

Q8.5   The following changes in isolation would tend to increase the result obtained in an ESR test:

A. an increase in the plasma viscosity from 1.50 cP to 2.00 cP.
B. a moderate decrease in the PCV.
C. cold agglutinins with a thermal amplitude up to 25°C.
D. an increase in the level of plasma fibrinogen.
E. marked spherocytosis.

Q8.6   The following statements relate to the ABO blood group system:

A. the soluble A and B antigens are glycoproteins.
B. the B antigen is formed by the addition of D-galactosamine to the H antigen.
C. the commonest subgroup of the A antigen is A_2.
D. the lectin derived from *Dolichos biflorus* agglutinates A_2 cells.
E. individuals with the "Bombay" phenotype typically express anti-H antibodies in their serum.

Q8.7   The following substances are important naturally-occurring inhibitors of coagulation *in vivo*:

A. antithrombin III (ATIII).
B. streptokinase.
C. ethylenediaminetetraacetic acid (EDTA).
D. heparin cofactor II   (HCII).
E. α_2-macroglobulin.

Q8.8   The following conditions are auto-immune disorders:

A. pernicious anaemia (PA).
B. paroxysmal cold haemoglobinuria (PCH).
C. systemic lupus erythematosis (SLE).
D. paroxysmal nocturnal haemoglobinuria (PNH).
E. Evans' syndrome.

A8.5   A. **True.** This would enhance rouleaux formation.
  B. **True.** This would reduce the packing effect of the sedimented red cells.
  C. **True.** The agglutinates settle rapidly.
  D. **True.** This would enhance rouleaux formation.
  E. **False.** Spherocytes do not pack efficiently.

Suggested Reading
  Hall and Malia, Chapter 7, Erythrocyte sedimentation rate, plasma viscosity and blood rheology.

A8.6   A. **True.**
  B. **False.** The B antigen is formed by the addition of D-galactose.
  C. **False.** A_1 is the commonest subgroup of A.
  D. **False.** *Dolichos biflorus* lectin has anti-A_1 specificity.
  E. **True.**

Suggested Reading
  Hoffbrand and Lewis, Chapter 9, Antigens in human blood.

A8.7   A. **True.**
  B. **False.** This substance is synthesised by streptococci. It is used therapeutically as a defibrinating agent.
  C. **False.** EDTA is an *in vitro* anticoagulant.
  D. **True.**
  E. **True.**

Suggested Reading
  Hoffbrand and Lewis, Chapter 21, Normal haemostasis.

A8.8   A. **True.** PA is associated with the formation of anti-parietal cell and anti-intrinsic factor auto-antibodies.
  B. **True.** PCH is an auto-immune haemolytic anaemia (AIHA).
  C. **True.** SLE is associated with a wide range of auto-antibodies.
  D. **False.** PNH is an acquired membrane abnormality.
  E. **True.** Evans' syndrome is the combination of AIHA with thrombocytopenia.

Suggested Reading
  Roitt, Brostoff and Male, Chapter 23, Autoimmunity and autoimmune disease.

Q8.9 **The following statements relate to the use of radio-isotopes in haematology:**

A. The SI unit of radioactivity is the becquerel (Bq).
B. The half-life of tritium (^{3}H) is very short.
C. The detector in most gamma counters is composed of sodium iodide.
D. The major source of error in gamma counting is colour quenching.
E. ^{111}In is a β particle emitter.

Q8.10 **Human erythropoietin**

A. is a phospholipid.
B. is normally present in the urine.
C. has a molecular weight of 34,000 daltons.
D. acts principally on pronormoblasts.
E. production is stimulated by tissue hypoxia.

Q8.11 **The following red cell membrane lipids are mainly present in the inner (cytosol) layer:**

A. sphingomyelin.
B. phosphatidyl serine.
C. unesterified cholesterol.
D. phosphatidyl ethanolamine.
E. phosphatidyl choline.

Q8.12 **The following conditions are primary platelet membrane defects:**

A. von Willebrand's disease.
B. pseudo-von Willebrand's disease.
C. Bernard-Soulier syndrome.
D. Grey platelet syndrome.
E. Glanzmann's thrombasthenia.

A8.9   A. **True.**   The becquerel is defined as 1 disintegration per second. The older unit was the curie (Ci).

  B. **False.**   The half-life of tritium is 12.3 years.

  C. **True.**

  D. **False.**   Colour quenching is associated with liquid scintillation counting of β particles.

  E. **False.** ^{111}In is a γ emitter.

Suggested Reading
Chanarin, Chapter 3, Radionuclides in haematology.

A8.10   A. **False.**   It is a glycoprotein.

  B. **True.**

  C. **True.**

  D. **False.**   It acts principally on BFU-E and CFU-E.

  E. **True.**

Suggested Reading
Hoffbrand and Lewis, Chapter 1, Erythropoiesis.

A8.11   A. **False.**   Sphingomyelin is mainly present in the outer layer.

  B. **True.**

  C. **False.**   Cholesterol is mainly present between the two layers.

  D. **True.**

  E. **False.**   Phosphatidyl choline is mainly present in the outer layer.

Suggested Reading
Hall and Malia, Chapter 2, Physiology of the blood.

A8.12   A. **False.**   VWD is a plasma defect.

  B. **True.**   This is caused by a defect of platelet glycoprotein Ib (GpIb) such that higher multimers of vWF are bound spontaneously.

  C. **True.**   This is caused by a deficiency of GpIb.

  D. **False.**   This is caused by deficiency of platelet α granules.

  E. **True.**   This is caused by a deficiency of GpIIb/IIIa.

Suggested Reading
Hoffbrand and Lewis, Chapter 22, Platelet disorders.

Q8.13 The following laboratory results are consistent with a diagnosis of severe type I von Willebrand's disease:

A. a factor VIII_c of 10 iu/dl.
B. a von Willebrand factor (vWF) of 100 iu/dl.
C. large multimers of vWF absent.
D. all tests of primary haemostasis normal.
E. platelet aggregation *in vitro* in response to adrenaline (epinephrine) normal.

Q8.14 The following laboratory results are characteristic of Waldenstrom's macroglobulinaemia

A. the abnormal cells form rosettes with sheep erythrocytes (E-rosettes).
B. the presence of a monoclonal IgG paraprotein in the serum.
C. blue background staining on Romanowsky-stained blood films.
D. a plasma viscosity at 25°C of 1.60 cP.
E. surface immunoglobulin (SIg) demonstrable on the abnormal cells by immunofluorescence.

Q8.15 The following features are characteristic of the blasts of L3 acute leukaemia:

A. Sudan black staining positive.
B. nucleoli are inconspicuous or absent.
C. intense cytoplasmic basophilia.
D. irregular nuclear shape with nuclear clefting.
E. markedly raised serum lysozyme level.

Q8.16 The following statements relate to deficiency of the enzyme glucose-6-phosphate dehydrogenase (G-6-PD):

A. individual red cells from female carriers all exhibit approximately 50% of normal activity.
B. favism is a recognised feature of the Mediterranean variant of the enzyme.
C. reticulocytes in male hemizygotes have higher levels of activity than their mature red cells.
D. Heinz bodies are a recognised feature of drug-induced haemolysis in G-6-PD deficient individuals.
E. the level of reduced glutathione is decreased in G-6-PD deficient individuals.

A8.13   A.   **True.**   The VIII$_c$ level falls because of the deficiency of vWF, its carrier protein.

       B.   **False.**   vWF synthesis is decreased in vWD.

       C.   **False.**

       D.   **False.**   Primary haemostasis typically is abnormal in vWD.

       E.   **True.**

Suggested Reading
Hall and Malia, Chapter 16, Haemorrhagic disorders.

A8.14   A.   **False.**   WM is a B cell disorder.

       B.   **False.**   The paraprotein is IgM.

       C.   **True.**   This is caused by the markedly increased plasma protein concentration.

       D.   **False.**   Plasma viscosity typically is markedly increased at diagnosis.

       E.   **True.**

Suggested Reading
Hoffbrand and Lewis, Chapter 18, Myelomatosis.

A8.15   A.   **False.**   ALL lymphoblasts are not stained by Sudan black.

       B.   **False.**   L3 lymphoblasts typically have at least one prominent nucleolus.

       C.   **True.**

       D.   **False.**   L3 lymphoblasts typically have regular oval or round nuclei.

       E.   **False.**   This is typical of M4.

Suggested Reading
Hall and Malia, Chapter 13, The proliferative disorders.

A8.16   A.   **False.**   Individual red cells from a heterozygote either have normal activity or are deficient.

       B.   **True.**

       C.   **True.**   G6-P-D activity decreases with increasing red cell age.

       D.   **True.**

       E.   **True.**

Suggested Reading
Hall and Malia, Chapter 11, Haemolytic anaemias.

Q8.17 The following abnormal haemoglobins result from β globin chain substitutions:

A. haemoglobin C.
B. haemoglobin D.
C. haemoglobin G Philadelphia.
D. haemoglobin Hammersmith.
E. haemoglobin Bristol.

Q8.18 The following statements relate to the malarial parasite *Plasmodium falciparum*:

A. the sexual phase of its life cycle occurs in man.
B. Wr^b negative red cells exhibit a markedly reduced susceptibility to invasion by the parasite.
C. red cells from heterozygotes for haemoglobin S sickle more readily when parasitised.
D. female carriers of glucose-6-phosphate dehydrogenase (G-6-PD) deficiency exhibit an increased resistance to this parasite.
E. the schizogonic cycle lasts 4 days.

Q8.19 The following statements relate to cytotoxic drugs:

A. busulphan (Myleran) is an alkylating agent.
B. cytosine arabinoside (Cytosar, Ara-C) is active only against cells in S phase of the cell cycle.
C. methotrexate acts as a competitive inhibitor of the enzyme dihydrofolate reductase.
D. vincristine (Oncovin) is derived from the Madagascar periwinkle (*Vinca rosea*).
E. folinic acid (Leucovorin) is used to "rescue" the bone marrow and mucosae from the acute toxicity of high dose methotrexate therapy.

Q8.20 Thrombomodulin

A. binds up to 4 molecules of thrombin per molecule of thrombomodulin.
B. has a molecular weight of 74,000 daltons.
C. acts as a cofactor in the activation of protein C.
D. exists bound to the outer membrane of vascular endothelial cells.
E. inactivates protein S *in vivo* by proteolysis.

A8.17 A. **True.** HbC is denoted β6(A3) glu–>lys.
B. **True.** HbD is denoted β121(GH4) glu–>gln.
C. **False.** HbG Philadelphia is denoted α68(E17) asn–>lys.
D. **True.** Hb Hammersmith is denoted
β42(CD1) phe–>ser.
E. **True.** Hb Bristol is denoted β67(E11) val–>asp.

Suggested Reading
Hall and Malia, Chapter 11, Haemolytic anaemias.

A8.18 A. **False.** Sporogeny occurs in the mosquito.
B. **True.** Susceptibility to invasion is reduced to about
10% of normal with this blood group.
C. **True.**
D. **True.** Parasites fail to develop within G-6-PD deficient
red cells.
E. **False.** Schizogony takes 48 h for *P. falciparum*.

Suggested Reading
Hall and Malia, Chapter 14, Haematology of infections.

A8.19 A. **True.** Busulphan acts by alkylating DNA which
interferes with replication and transcription.
B. **True.** Ara-C is a pyrimidine analogue.
C. **True.**
D. **True.**
E. **True.**

Suggested Reading
Hoffbrand and Lewis, Chapter 14, Acute leukaemia.

A8.20 A. **False.** One molecule of thrombin is bound per molecule
of thrombomodulin.
B. **True.**
C. **True.** The thrombin:thrombomodulin complex
potentiates activation of protein C by several
thousand times.
D. **True.**
E. **False.**

Suggested Reading
Hoffbrand and Lewis, Chapter 21, Normal haemostasis.

Multiple Choice Test Nine

Q9.1   The mean red cell volume (MCV)

A. typically is increased in severe vitamin B_{12} deficiency.
B. typically is increased in homozygous β^+ thalassaemia.
C. is derived using the formula PCV x MCH.
D. increases in mildly hypotonic suspending fluids.
E. typically is increased in chronic alcohol abuse.

Q9.2   The following laboratory results are normal for an adult female:

A. an absolute eosinophil count of $0.2 \times 10^9/l$.
B. a serum vitamin B_{12} level of 400 pg/l.
C. a plasma viscosity at 25°C of 1.60 cP.
D. a serum ferritin of 30 ng/l.
E. a packed cell volume (PCV) of 0.40.

Q9.3   The following conditions are established triggers of disseminated intravascular coagulation (DIC):

A. abruptio placentae.
B. meningococcal septicaemia
C. amniotic fluid embolism.
D. hydatidiform mole.
E. M3 leukaemia.

Q9.4   The following cells are capable of mitosis:

A. neutrophil metamyelocyte.
B. reticulocyte.
C. eosinophil.
D. promyelocyte.
E. T lymphocyte.

A9.1 A. **True.** Megaloblastic anaemias typically are macrocytic.
        B. **False.** The thalassaemias typically are microcytic.
        C. **False.** MCV = PCV/RBC.
        D. **True.** Suspension in hypotonic media causes the red cell to absorb water to restore tonicity.
        E. **True.** Alcohol has a direct toxic effect on the bone marrow and also leads to liver damage. Both of these can result in macrocytosis.

Suggested Reading
Eastham, Chapter 3, Anaemia.

A9.2 A. **True.** The normal range is 0.04-0.4 x 10^9/l.
        B. **False.** The normal range is 170-970 ng/l.
        C. **True.** The normal range is 1.50-1.72 cP.
        D. **False.** The normal range is 30-185 µg/l.
        E. **True.** The normal range is 0.36-0.47.

Suggested Reading
Hall and Malia, Chapter 2, Physiology of the blood.

A9.3 A. **True.**
        B. **True.**
        C. **True.**
        D. **True.**
        E. **True.**

Suggested Reading
Hall and Malia, Chapter 16, Haemorrhagic disorders.

A9.4 A. **False.** By this stage, the neutrophil has lost the capacity for division.
        B. **False.** The reticulocyte has no nucleus.
        C. **False.** Mature eosinophils are end-stage cells.
        D. **True.**
        E. **True.**

Suggested Reading
Hall and Malia, Chapter 1, Haemopoiesis.

Q9.5   The following findings are consistent with a diagnosis of myeloma:

A. marked rouleaux formation on the blood film.
B. marked hypocalcaemia.
C. leucoerythroblastic blood picture.
D. widespread osteolytic lesions.
E. a polyclonal increase in serum immunoglobulins.

Q9.6   The following red cell inclusions contain iron:

A. Pappenheimer bodies.
B. Howell-Jolly bodies.
C. Heinz bodies.
D. Cabot's rings.
E. punctate basophilia.

Q9.7   The following blood changes characteristically are present two weeks post-splenectomy in the absence of haematological disease:

A. absolute neutrophil leucocytosis.
B. Howell-Jolly bodies in some red cells.
C. circulating siderocytes.
D. absolute thrombocytosis.
E. increased osmotic fragility.

Q9.8   The following statements relate to different forms of autoimmune haemolytic anaemia (AIHA):

A. methyldopa (Aldomet) induces haemolysis by the "innocent bystander" mechanism.
B. the Donath-Landsteiner antibody typically is IgM.
C. warm AIHA is more common than cold AIHA.
D. the Donath-Landsteiner antibody typically has anti-I specificity.
E. in paroxysmal cold haemoglobinuria (PCH), haemolysis can be demonstrated at 4°C.

A9.5   A. **True.**   Rouleaux formation is induced by the increased plasma protein concentration.

  B. **False.**   Hypercalcaemia secondary to osteolysis is more usually seen.

  C. **True.**   About 10% of cases at diagnosis have a leucoerythroblastic blood picture.

  D. **True.**   More than 50% of cases at diagnosis have some degree of osteolysis.

  E. **False.**   The paraprotein is monoclonal.

Suggested Reading
Hoffbrand and Lewis, Chapter 18, Myelomatosis.

A9.6   A. **True.**   Pappenheimer bodies are siderotic granules.

  B. **False.**   Howell Jolly bodies are nuclear remnants.

  C. **True.**   Heinz bodies consist of denatured haemoglobin.

  D. **True.**   Cabot's rings contain both iron and histone although their precise nature remains uncertain.

  E. **False.**   Punctate basophilia represents aggregated ribosomes.

Suggested Reading
Eastham, Chapter 2, Red blood cells.

A9.7   A. **True.**   The post-operative neutrophil leucocytosis can last for several weeks.

  B. **True.**   These nuclear remnants are normally removed by the spleen.

  C. **True.**

  D. **True.**   The thrombocytosis typically peaks about two weeks post-splenectomy.

  E. **False.**   Osmotic fragility typically is decreased.

Suggested Reading
Hoffbrand and Lewis, Chapter 1, Erythropoiesis.

A9.8   A. **False.**   Methyldopa induces autoantibody formation in affected individuals.

  B. **False.**   The D-L antibody is IgG.

  C. **True.**   Warm AIHA is about 4 times more common.

  D. **False.**   The D-L antibody typically has anti-P specificity.

  E. **False.**   Sensitisation occurs at 4°C, haemolysis at 37°C.

Suggested Reading
Hoffbrand and Lewis, Chapter 7, Acquired haemolytic anaemias.

Q9.9   **Lupus anticoagulant**

A. typically results in a severe bleeding tendency.
B. is an antibody directed against anionic phospholipid.
C. is only found in patients with systemic lupus
   erythematosis (SLE).
D. is a recognised cause of recurrent spontaneous abortion.
E. typically causes prolongation of the APTT.

Q9.10   **The following conditions are primary platelet disorders:**

A. Gaisbock's syndrome.
B. Henoch-Schönlein purpura.
C. Glanzmann's thrombasthenia.
D. senile purpura.
E. Bernard-Soulier syndrome.

Q9.11   **The following statements relate to protein S:**

A. it is present in platelet α granules.
B. its activity is enhanced when it is bound to $C4_b$.
C. it inactivates protein C irreversibly by forming a complex
   with it.
D. plasma activity is decreased by effective
   warfarin therapy.
E. its activity is greatly enhanced by thrombin cleavage.

Q9.12   **The following statements relate to the life cycle of
malarial parasites:**

A. sporogeny only occurs in mammals.
B. they are carried by a number of species of sandfly of the
   genus *Phlebotomus*.
C. infected mosquitoes inject both male and female
   gametocytes into humans while feeding.
D. schizonts are most frequently seen in samples taken at the
   peak of pyrexia.
E. the male gametocytes characteristically are
   larger than the female gametocytes.

A9.9 A. **False.** Lupus anticoagulant typically predisposes to venous thrombosis.
B. **True.**
C. **False.** It is found in association with a variety of connective tissue disorders.
D. **True.** This is often the presenting feature.
E. **True.**

Suggested Reading
Hoffbrand and Lewis, Chapter 24, Acquired disorders of haemostasis.

A9.10 A. **False.** Gaisbock's syndrome is a relative polycythaemia.
B. **False.** HSP is an allergic vasculitis.
C. **True.** Glanzmann's thrombasthenia is due to deficiency of platelet glycoproteins IIb/IIIa.
D. **False.** Senile purpura results from atrophy of collagen in blood vessels.
E. **True.** Bernard Soulier syndrome results from deficiency of platelet glycoprotein Ib.

Suggested Reading
Hoffbrand and Lewis, Chapter 22, Platelet disorders.

A9.11 A. **False.**
B. **False.** The bound form of protein S is inactive.
C. **False.** It is a cofactor of the anticoagulant activity of protein C.
D. **True.** It is vitamin K-dependent.
E. **False.** Thrombin-cleaved protein S inhibits the anticoagulant activity of protein C.

Suggested Reading
Hoffbrand and Lewis, Chapter 21, Normal haemostasis.

A9.12 A. **False.** Sporogeny is restricted to the mosquito.
B. **False.** Malarial parasites are carried by the *Anopheles* mosquito. *Phlebotomus* sandflies carry *Leishmania donovani*.
C. **False.** Sporozoites are injected during feeding.
D. **False.** Schizonts are rare at this time; early trophozoites are the most common stage seen.
E. **False.** Male gametocytes typically are smaller.

Suggested Reading
Hall and Malia, Chapter 14, Haematology of infections

Q9.13 The following differentiation antigens are markers of T lymphocytes:

A. CD22.
B. CD1.
C. CD4.
D. CD19.
E. CD14.

Q9.14 Plasma haptoglobins

A. bind free α globin chains avidly.
B. are synthesised in the liver.
C. are glycoproteins.
D. are usually absent from cord blood.
E. typically are decreased in paroxysmal nocturnal haemoglobinuria (PNH).

Q9.15 Urinary excretion of coproporphyrin characteristically is increased in the following conditions:

A. hereditary protoporphyria.
B. iron deficiency anaemia.
C. lead poisoning.
D. erythropoietic porphyria.
E. porphyria cutanea tarda.

Q9.16 The following statements relate to the structure of the human β globin gene:

A. the polyadenylation (polyA) signal is located at the $5'$ end of the gene.
B. it is composed of 4 exons and 3 introns.
C. the TATA promoter box is located about 30 bp upstream (ie towards the $5'$ end) from the gene.
D. the exon-intron junctions are characterised by the dinucleotides GT ($5'$) and AG ($3'$).
E. transcription of the gene begins at the $3'$ end.

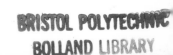

A9.13   A.   **False.**   CD22 is a B lymphocyte marker.

        B.   **True.**   CD1 is a marker of cortical thymocytes.

        C.   **True.**   CD4 is a marker of T helper cells.

        D.   **False.**   CD19 is a pan B lymphocyte marker.

        E.   **False.**   CD14 is a marker of monocyte/macrophage and myeloid cells.

Suggested Reading

Chanarin, Chapter 11, Immunological markers.

A9.14   A.   **False.**   Haptoglobin does not bind free α chains.

        B.   **True.**

        C.   **True.**

        D.   **True.**

        E.   **True.**   Haptoglobin levels are decreased in cases of intravascular haemolysis.

Suggested Reading

Hall and Malia, Chapter 2, Physiology of the blood.

A9.15   A.   **False.**   This disorder is due to deficiency of haem synthetase. The excess porphyrin is excreted exclusively in the faeces.

        B.   **True.**

        C.   **True.**   Urinary coproporphyrin is markedly increased in lead poisoning.

        D.   **True.**   This disorder is due to deficiency of uroporphyrinogen cosynthetase.

        E.   **True.**   This is the commonest of the porphyrias and is due to deficiency of hepatic uroporphyrinogen decarboxylase.

Suggested Reading

Hoffbrand and Lewis, Chapter 2, Iron.

A9.16   A.   **False.**   The polyA signal is located $3'$ of the gene.

        B.   **False.**   It contains 3 exons and 2 introns.

        C.   **True.**

        D.   **True.**   These dinucleotides are an absolute requirement for splicing of the introns.

        E.   **False.**   Transcription occurs $5' \rightarrow 3'$.

Suggested Reading

Hoffbrand and Lewis, Chapter 5, The haemoglobinopathies.

Q9.17 The following laboratory results are consistent with a diagnosis of sickle cell disease which is not in crisis:

A. absolute reticulocytopenia.
B. a ^{51}Cr-determined mean cell lifespan (MCL) of 25 days.
C. the presence of a single band cathodic to the haemoglobin A standard on tris-EDTA-borate electrophoresis at pH 8.4.
D. the presence of a band anodic to haemoglobin A standard on citrate agar electrophoresis at pH 6.2.
E. a shortened time in the acidified glycerol lysis test (AGLT$_{50}$).

Q9.18 The following haemoglobins have a higher oxygen affinity than haemoglobin A:

A. haemoglobin F ($\alpha_2\gamma_2$).
B. haemoglobin Chesapeake (α(FG4) arg—>leu).
C. haemoglobin H (β_4).
D. haemoglobin Barts (γ_4).
E. haemoglobin Kansas (β(G4) asp—>thr).

Q9.19 Urinary erythropoietin levels typically are increased in the following conditions:

A. polycythaemia rubra vera (PRV).
B. Blackfan Diamond syndrome.
C. chronic renal failure (CRF).
D. haemoglobin Chesapeake disease.
E. chronic pulmonary insufficiency.

A9.17 A. **False.** Reticulocytes typically are increased.
        B. **True.**   The normal MCL is 120 days.
        C. **True.**   Further tests are required to identify the band
                         as HbS.
        D. **True.**   See C.
        E. **False.** This is consistent with hereditary spherocytosis.

Suggested Reading
Hall and Malia, Chapter 11, Haemolytic anaemias.

A9.18 A. **True.**   This facilitates the transfer of oxygen from the
                         maternal to the foetal circulation *in utero*.
        B. **True.**
        C. **True.**
        D. **True.**
        E. **False.** Hb Kansas is a low-affinity haemoglobin.

Suggested Reading
Eastham, Chapter 1, Haemoglobin and associated pigments.

A9.19 A. **False.** Urinary EPO levels are normal or decreased
                         in PRV.
        B. **True.**   This is pure red cell aplasia: EPO is released
                         secondary to tissue hypoxia.
        C. **False.** Urinary EPO levels typically are low in CRF.
        D. **True.**   Hb Chesapeake is a high oxygen affinity
                         haemoglobin which is associated with secondary
                         polycythaemia due to tissue hypoxia.
        E. **True.**   Pulmonary insufficiency induces EPO release
                         secondary to tissue hypoxia.

Suggested Reading
Eastham, Chapter 2, Red blood cells.

Q9.20 **The following statements relate to the molecular biology of of factor VIII$_c$.**

A. the gene contains 3 exons and 2 introns.
B. the restriction endonuclease Taq I recognises several "hot-spots" for point mutation within the gene.
C. partial gene deletions are always associated with the development of an inhibitor.
D. the intragenic Bgl I restriction fragment length polymorphism (RFLP) is particularly useful for determination of haemophilia carrier status in American blacks.
E. the carrier status of all females can be accurately determined using intragenic RFLP analysis.

A9.20 A. **False.** It contains 26 exons and 25 introns.
  B. **True.** Taq I recognises the sequence TCGA. C-T mutations are relatively common due to methylation and subsequent spontaneous deamination.
  C. **False.** There is no apparent relationship between deletion size or position and the development of inhibitors in haemophilia A.
  D. **True.** This RFLP is adjacent to exon 26.
  E. **False.** Only about 70% of European females are currently informative using this technique.

Suggested Reading

Hoffbrand and Lewis, Chapter 23, Inherited bleeding disorders.

Multiple Choice Test Ten

Q10.1 **Absolute eosinophilia is a recognised feature of**

A. parasitic helminthic infestation eg schistosomiasis.
B. psoriasis.
C. hay fever.
D. asthma.
E. aplastic anaemia.

Q10.2 **The following laboratory results are normal for a neonate:**

A. mean cell volume (MCV) of 105 fl.
B. a reticulocyte count of 5%.
C. an absolute neutrophil count of 5.0×10^9/l.
D. an absolute lymphocyte count of 1.5×10^9/l.
E. a haemoglobin level of 15.0 g/dl.

Q10.3 **The following substances are red cell membrane cytoskeletal proteins:**

A. spectrin.
B. fibronectin.
C. ankyrin.
D. actin.
E. β_2 microglobulin.

Q10.4 **von Willebrand factor (vWF)**

A. is coded for by a gene on the X chromosome.
B. is synthesised by vascular endothelial cells.
C. binds platelets to vascular endothelium at sites of vascular damage.
D. is reduced or absent in haemophilia A.
E. is present in platelet α granules.

Q10.5 **The following statements relate to Intrinsic Factor (IF):**

A. it is synthesised mainly in the terminal ileum.
B. it is essential for the absorption of dietary folate.
C. it is a phospholipid.
D. it has a molecular weight of 114,000 daltons.
E. its production is stimulated by the presence of histamine.

A10.1 A. **True.**
        B. **True.**
        C. **True.**
        D. **True.**
        E. **False.**

Suggested Reading
Eastham, Chapter 4, Peripheral white blood cells.

A10.2 A. **True.**   The normal range is 100-115 fl.
        B. **True.**   The normal range is 2-6%.
        C. **False.** The normal range is $6.0\text{-}14.0 \times 10^9/\text{l}$.
        D. **False.** The normal range is $2.5\text{-}5.0 \times 10^9/\text{l}$.
        E. **True.**   The normal range is 13.6-19.6 g/dl.

Suggested Reading
Hall and Malia, Chapter 2, Physiology of the blood.

A10.3 A. **True.**
        B. **False.** Fibronectin is an adhesive plasma protein.
        C. **True.**
        D. **True.**
        E. **False.** β_2 microglobulin is a polypeptide which is associated with HLA class I antigens.

Suggested Reading
Hall and Malia, Chapter 2, Physiology of the blood.

A10.4 A. **False.** VWF is coded for on the p arm of chromosome number 12.
        B. **True.**   It is also synthesised by megakaryocytes.
        C. **True.**
        D. **False.** VIII_c is reduced in haemophilia A.
        E. **True.**

Suggested Reading
Hoffbrand and Lewis, Chapter 21, Normal haemostasis.

A10.5 A. **False.** It is synthesised by gastric parietal cells.
        B. **False.** It is required for vitamin B_{12} absorption.
        C. **False.** It is a glycoprotein.
        D. **True.**
        E. **True.**

Suggested Reading
Hoffbrand and Lewis, Chapter 3, Megaloblastic anaemia.

Q10.6 The following conditions are vasculopathies:

A. senile purpura.
B. Henoch-Schönlein purpura.
C. pseudo-von Willebrand's disease.
D. hereditary haemorrhagic telangiectasia (HHT).
E. Ehlers-Danlos syndrome.

Q10.7 The following statements relate to red blood cell enzymopathies:

A. deficiency of glucose-6-phosphate dehydrogenase (G-6-PD) is inherited as an autosomal recessive disorder.
B. pyruvate kinase deficiency is most common in countries where malaria is endemic.
C. the most common defect of the Embden-Meyerhof pathway is hexokinase deficiency.
D. deficiency of pyrimidine 5' nucleotidase is strongly associated with prominent basophilic stippling.
E. favism is most commonly seen in the presence of Gd^{A-} G-6-PD deficiency.

Q10.8 The following substances are important naturally-occurring inhibitors of coagulation *in vivo*:

A. antithrombin III (ATIII).
B. streptokinase.
C. ethylenediaminetetraacetic acid (EDTA).
D. heparin cofactor II (HCII).
E. α_2-macroglobulin.

Q10.9 The following statements relate to haemoglobins produced *in utero* in health and disease:

A. haemoglobin Portland has the composition $\zeta_2\gamma_2$.
B. haemoglobin Gower I has the composition ε_4.
C. haemoglobin Gower II has the composition $\alpha_2\varepsilon_2$.
D. haemoglobin Barts has the composition β_4.
E. haemoglobin H has the composition γ_4.

A10.6   A. **True.**   Senile purpura results from atrophy of collagen.
     B. **True.**   HSP is an allergic vasculitis.
     C. **False.**   Pseudo-vWD is a platelet defect.
     D. **True.**   HHT is characterised by capillary fragility and malformation.
     E. **True.**   Ehlers-Danlos syndrome is a disorder of connective tissue.

Suggested Reading
Hall and Malia, Chapter 16, Haemorrhagic disorders.

A10.7   A. **False.**   G-6-PD deficiency is inherited as an X-linked recessive disorder.
     B. **False.**   The incidence of PK deficiency is unrelated to that of malaria.
     C. **False.**   PK deficiency is the most common defect.
     D. **True.**
     E. **False.**   Favism is associated with the isoenzymes Gd^{Med} and Gd^{Canton}.

Suggested Reading
Hoffbrand and Lewis, Chapter 6, Inherited haemolytic anaemias.

A10.8   A. **True.**
     B. **False.**   This substance is synthesised by streptococci. It is used therapeutically as a defibrinating agent.
     C. **False.**   EDTA is an *in vitro* anticoagulant.
     D. **True.**
     E. **True.**

A10.9   A. **True.**
     B. **False.**   Hb Gower I has the composition $\zeta_2\varepsilon_2$.
     C. **True.**
     D. **False.**   Hb Barts has the composition γ_4.
     E. **False.**   HbH has the composition β_4.

Suggested Reading
Hall and Malia, Chapter 1, Haemopoiesis,
Hall and Malia, Chapter 9, Microcytic anaemias.

Q10.10 The level of 2,3-diphosphoglycerate (2,3-DPG) typically is decreased in the following conditions:

A. normal, uncomplicated pregnancy.
B. pyruvate kinase (PK) deficiency.
C. in donor blood after 3 weeks storage at 4°C.
D. severe hexokinase deficiency.
E. lactic acidosis.

Q10.11 The following statements relate to the electrophoretic mobilities of haemoglobin variants at pH 6.0:

A. haemoglobins S and D do not separate.
B. haemoglobin F migrates towards the cathode.
C. haemoglobins D and G do not separate.
D. haemoglobin C migrates towards the anode.
E. haemoglobin O^{Arab} does not separate from haemoglobin E.

Q10.12 Platelet dense granules contain the following substances:

A. platelet factor 4.
B. platelet factor 1.
C. 5-hydroxytryptamine (serotonin).
D. myeloperoxidase.
E. acetylsalicylic acid.

Q10.13 The following laboratory results are characteristic of polycythaemia rubra vera (PRV) in a 80 kg man:

A. a plasma volume of 2,400 ml.
B. a venous packed cell volume of 0.58.
C. a total red cell volume (TRCV) of 2,500 ml.
D. a leucocyte alkaline phosphatase (LAP) score of 11/100 neutrophils.
E. a splenic red cell volume of 400 ml.

A10.10 A. **False.** 2,3-DPG levels typically are raised during pregnancy.
   B. **False.** Pyruvate kinase acts below the Rappaport-Luebering shunt and so deficiency leads to an accumulation of 2,3-DPG.
   C. **True.** The decreased level of 2,3-DPG is due to failure of glycolysis in stored blood.
   D. **True.** Hexokinase acts above the Rappaport-Luebering shunt.
   E. **True.**

Suggested Reading
Eastham, Chapter 1, Haemoglobin and related pigments.

A10.11 A. **False.** HbS migrates anodically to HbD.
   B. **True.**
   C. **True.**
   D. **True.**
   E. **False.** HbO^{Arab} migrates anodically to HbE.

Suggested Reading
Hall and Malia, Chapter 11, Haemolytic anaemias.

A10.12 A. **False.** PF4 is a constituent of α granules.
   B. **False.** PF1 is a constituent of α granules.
   C. **True.**
   D. **False.** Myeloperoxidase is a constituent of neutrophil primary granules.
   E. **False.** Aspirin is normally absent.

Suggested Reading
Hoffbrand and Lewis, Chapter 21, Normal haemostasis.

A10.13 A. **False.** Plasma volume typically is normal.
   B. **True.**
   C. **False.** The TRCV must be greater than 36 ml/kg for a diagnosis of PRV in an adult male.
   D. **False.** The LAP score typically is raised in PRV.
   E. **True.** The normal range is 70-80 ml.

Suggested Reading
Hoffbrand and Lewis, Chapter 20, Non-leukaemic myeloproliferative disorders.

Q10.14 Red cells from the following species are agglutinated by the heterophil antibody present in the serum of a patient suffering from glandular fever:

A. sheep.
B. guinea-pig.
C. horse.
D. rat.
E. ox.

Q10.15 Human IgM immunoglobulin

A. is the source of passive immunity in babies by placental transfer.
B. is concerned mainly with the primary antibody response.
C. exists as a pentamer.
D. is present in high concentration in extravascular fluid.
E. accounts for 70-80% of serum immunoglobulins.

Q10.16 The following laboratory results are characteristic of haemoglobin H disease (α-/--):

A. 1% haemoglobin Barts in the cord blood.
B. a raised haemoglobin F level in an adult.
C. basophilic stippling on the blood film.
D. 40% haemoglobin H in the cord blood.
E. marked microcytosis and hypochromia on the blood film.

Q10.17 The following statements relate to the action of cytotoxic drugs used in leukaemia chemotherapy:

A. 6-mercaptopurine is a pyrimidine antagonist.
B. chlorambucil (Leukeran) is an alkylating agent.
C. cytosine arabinoside (Cytosar, Ara-C) is a pyrimidine antagonist.
D. vincristine (Oncovin) inhibits mitotic spindle formation.
E. methotrexate is a purine antagonist.

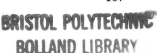

A10.14 A. **True.**
B. **False.**
C. **True.**
D. **False.**
E. **True.**

Suggested Reading
Hall and Malia, Chapter 14, Haematology of infections.

A10.15 A. **False.** IgM cannot cross the placental barrier.
B. **True.**
C. **True.**
D. **False.** IgM does not leave the vascular space.
E. **False.** 70-80% of serum immunoglobulins are IgG.

Suggested Reading
Hoffbrand and Lewis, Chapter 8, Blood group serology.

A10.16 A. **False.** The cord blood contains about 25% Hb Barts.
B. **False.** This is suggestive of β thalassaemia.
C. **True.**
D. **False.** The cord blood contains 5-25% HbH.
E. **True.**

Suggested Reading
Hall and Malia, Chapter 9, Microcytic anaemias.

A10.17 A. **False.** 6-MP is a purine analogue.
B. **True.**
C. **True.**
D. **True.**
E. **False.** MTX is a folate analogue.

Suggested Reading
Hoffbrand and Lewis, Chapter 14, Acute leukaemia.

Q10.18 **The following statements relate to human T-lymphotropic retrovirus I (HTLV-I):**

A. it is causally related to chronic lymphocytic leukaemia (CLL) in Japan.
B. it contains the cell-derived oncogene c-myc.
C. it is used to immortalise cord blood T cells in *in vitro* culture.
D. a related virus, HTLV II, can be isolated from most cases of hairy cell leukaemia.
E. it is causally related to acquired immunodeficiency syndrome (AIDS).

Q10.19 **The following abnormal haemoglobins are designated as unstable variants:**

A. haemoglobin Hyde Park (β 92 (F8) his—>tyr).
B. haemoglobin Köln (β 98 (FG5) val—>meth).
C. haemoglobin G Philadelphia (α 68 (E17) asn—>lys).
D. haemoglobin Hammersmith (β42(CD1) phe—>ser).
E. haemoglobin Sabine (β 19 (F7) leu—>pro).

Q10.20 **The following haemopoietic growth factors are coded for on the stated chromosomes:**

A. interleukin-3 (IL-3) on the X chromosome.
B. granulocyte macrophage colony stimulating factor (GM-CSF) on chromosome 5.
C. granulocyte colony stimulating factor (G-CSF) on chromosome 7.
D. macrophage colony stimulating factor (M-CSF) on chromosome 17.
E. erythropoietin on chromosome 5.

A10.18 A. **False.** HTLV-I is implicated in a variant of T ALL which is seen most frequently in Japan and in the Caribbean.

B. **False.** It does not contain any cell-derived oncogene.

C. **True.**

D. **False.** HTLV-II has only been isolated from the rare T cell variant of HCL.

E. **False.** HIV is the causative agent of AIDS.

Suggested Reading

Roitt, Brostoff and Male, Chapter 16, Immunity to viruses, bacteria and fungi.

Recent advances in haematology 4, Chapter 9, Viruses, *onc* genes and leukaemia.

A10.19 A. **False.** Hb Hyde Park is one of the HbMs.

B. **True.** Hb Köln results from substitution of a haem contact amino acid.

C. **False.**

D. **True.** Hb Hammersmith results from substitution of a haem contact amino acid.

E. **True.** Hb Sabine results from substitution of proline in a helical portion of the molecule.

Suggested Reading

Hall and Malia, Chapter 11, Haemolytic anaemias.

A10.20 A. **False.** IL-3 is coded for on chromosome 5.

B. **True.**

C. **False.** G-CSF is coded for on chromosome 17.

D. **False.** M-CSF is coded for on chromosome 5.

E. **False.** EPO is coded for on chromosome 7.

Suggested Reading

Recent advances in haematology 5, Chapter 1, Haemopoietic growth factors: *in vitro* and *in vivo* studies.

Part Two
Case Studies

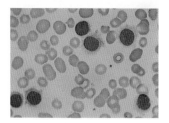

Plate 1 Blood film from case 1

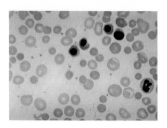

Plate 2 Blood film from case 2*

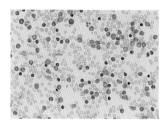

Plate 3 Blood film from case 3

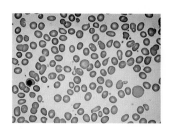

Plate 4 Blood film from case 5*

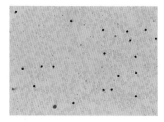

Plate 5 Blood film from case 6

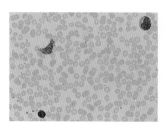

Plate 6 Blood film from case 7

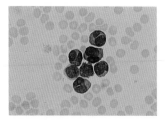

Plate 7 Blood film from case 8

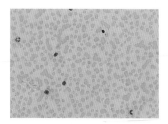

Plate 8 Blood film from case 10

*The blood films for cases 2,5,13 and 22 have been reproduced from A.V. Hoffbrand and J.E. Pettit (Eds). (1987). Slide Atlas of Clinical Haematology. London: Gower Medical with permission.

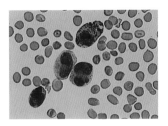

Plate 9 Blood film from case 11

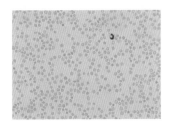

Plate 10 Blood film from case 12

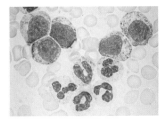

Plate 11 Blood film from case 13*

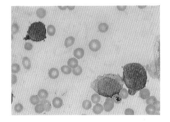

Plate 12 Blood film from case 15

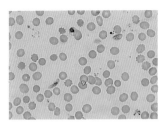

Plate 13 Blood film from case 16

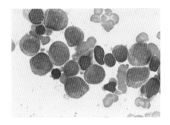

Plate 14 Blood film from case 18

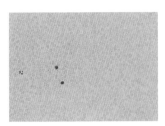

Plate 15 Blood film from case 21

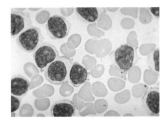

Plate 16 Blood film from case 22*

Introduction

The twenty-five case studies and related questions which are included in this section are designed to test interpretative skills as well as general knowledge of haematology. Each consists of brief clinical details relating to the presentation and clinical history of the patient as well as the results of the laboratory investigation. The range of disease states included does not reflect any particular balance between red cell and white cell disorders or malignant and non-malignant disorders.

None of the information is included to deliberately mislead, although not all is directly relevant or helpful. In each case, however, several clues to the most likely diagnosis are present.

The initial task in each case is to suggest the most likely diagnosis. A conclusion should only be reached after careful consideration of *all* of the relevant information. The most likely diagnoses are given on pages 166-167. These are provided separately to the answers to the other questions because, in some cases, it is important to know the diagnosis before answering the remaining questions. Thus, the diagnosis should be confirmed before proceeding to the other questions.

Colour plates of the blood films of certain cases are shown between pages 112 and 113. Refer to these before reaching a conclusion on the most likely diagnosis.

The questions to these case studies are not graded in the manner of the multiple choice tests in Part One of this book. No marks should be deducted for incorrect answers. As before, a good HNC/D student should score an average of 40% over a series of case studies, while a final FIMLS student should expect to score consistently above 80%.

The suggested reading is selected from the short list shown in the introduction to the multiple choice tests and should be used in the manner described there.

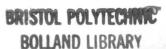

Case 1

Clinical Details

A 58-year-old man presented to his general practitioner complaining of general debility, fatigue and a persistent sore throat.

Clinical examination revealed moderate pallor and a moderately enlarged spleen. There was no enlargement of the lymph nodes.

Blood samples were obtained for analysis. The results are shown below. The full blood count was processed on a Technicon H*1.

Laboratory Results

WBC scattergram

CBC		
H	15.34	$\times 10^9$/l	WBC
L	2.55	$\times 10^{12}$/l	RBC
L	8.3	g/dl	HGB
L	21.5	%	HCT
	84.9	fl	MCV
	32.5	pg	MCH
	38.6	g/dl	MCHC
	18.9	%	RDW
	2.11	g/dl	HDW
	209	$\times 10^9$/l	PLT
	7.3	fl	MPV
	52.2	%	PDW
	.18	%	PCT

	%	DIFF		$\times 10^9$/l
L	10.6	NEUT	L	1.63
	43.3	LYMP	H	6.64
	1.4	MONO		.21
	.2	EOS		.03
	.2	BASO		.03
H	44.3	LUC	H	6.80
LI				2.33
MPXI				.9

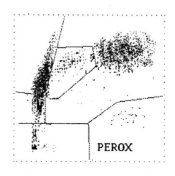

PEROX

Blood film report

Absolute lymphocytosis with many atypical forms present. Many lymphocytes show ragged cytoplasm.

The blood film from this patient is shown in Plate 1.

Cytochemistry

Acid Phosphatase +++
Ac. Phos. + Tartrate +++

Questions

Q1.1 What is the most likely diagnosis in this case?

Q1.2 What is the significance of the tartrate-resistant acid phosphatase (TRAP) activity?

Q1.3 What are LUC's?

Q1.4 What is the cause of the high LUC count in this case?

Q1.5 Complete the following table for this condition.

Male : female ratio
TRAP   +++
SmIg
E-rosettes
PAS
α-naphthyl butyrate esterase
β-glucuronidase
CD5
CD10
CD22
CD25

Mark the following True or False.

Q1.6 The following are recognised as useful in the successful treatment of this disorder?

    A. melphalan
    B. desferrioxamine
    C. splenectomy
    D. total body irradiation
    E. interferon-α
    F. plasmapheresis
    G. $2'$-deoxycoformycin

Case 2

Clinical Details

During a routine domiciliary visit by the district midwife, mild jaundice was noted in an otherwise healthy 5-day-old baby boy. No obvious jaundice had been present 48 hours after delivery when mother and baby were discharged.

The mother was 16 years old and this was her first pregnancy. She had been in good health throughout the pregnancy and the delivery had been uneventful.

Blood samples were obtained from both mother and baby for investigation. The results are shown below. The full blood count for the baby was processed on a Coulter S+IV.

Laboratory Results

WBC	14.6	R1
LY%	74.7	
MO%	7.2	
GR%	18.1	
LY#	10.9	R1
MO#	1.1	R1
GR#	2.6	R1
RBC	4.10	
HGB	14.6	
HCT	44.7	
MCV	109.0	H
MCH	35.6	
MCHC	32.7	
RDW	18.8	
PLT	335	
PCT	.275	
MPV	8.2	
PDW	13.3	

Blood film report

ANI	+
POLY	+
SPHERO	+

Occasional nucleated RBC seen.

The blood film from this baby is shown in Plate 2.

Serum bilirubin (baby)
19 µmol/l (NR 5-17 µmol/l)

Serology

	Mother	Baby
anti-A$_1$	-	+
anti-B	-	-
anti-D	-	+
anti-C	-	+
anti-E	-	-
anti-c	+	+
anti-e	+	+
DAG	-	+

IAT on heat eluate of baby cells
A$_1$ cells +
B cells -

Maternal serum antibody titre
IgG anti-A 1/32,000
IgG anti-B 1/8,000

Questions

Q2.1 What is the most likely diagnosis in this case?

Q2.2 What is the likely prognosis for the baby?

Q2.3 What is the risk of this disorder occurring in subsequent pregnancies?

Q2.4 Complete the following table.

Genotype		Frequency in UK population (%)
R_1r	CDe/cde	31
R_1R_1		
rr		
R_1R_2		
R_2r		
R_2R_2		

Q2.5 From the results shown, what are the most likely rhesus genotypes of the mother and her baby?

Q2.6 Complete the following table.

Lectin	Blood group specificity
Dolichos biflorus	
Ulex europaeus	
Vicia graminea	
Helix pomatia	
Fomes fomentarius	

Case 3

Clinical Details

A 10-month-old Cypriot boy was taken to his general practitioner by his parents because of lassitude and failure to thrive.

Clinical examination revealed an underweight child with poor muscular development, moderate pallor and a swollen abdomen due to splenomegaly. There was no lymphadenopathy.

The child had two sisters, both of whom were in good health. A careful family history revealed that two of the child's cousins in Cyprus had died before the age of four.

Blood samples were obtained for analysis. The results are shown below. The full blood count was processed on a Coulter S+IV.

Laboratory Results

Cell volume histogram

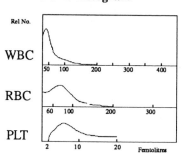

WBC	58.8	H	
LY%	76.6	H	R1
MO%	1.3		R1
GR%	22.1	L	R1
LY#	45.0	H	R1
MO#	.8		R1
GR#	13.0		R1
RBC	3.99		
HGB	7.0	L	
HCT	23.2	L	
MCV	58.2	L	
MCH	17.5	L	
MCHC	30.1		
RDW	24.6	H	
PLT	....		
PCT	....		
MPV	....		
PDW	....		

Blood film report

ANISO   +++
POIK   +++
MICRO   ++
HYPO   ++
TAR ++

Basophilic stippling prominent.
385 nucleated RBC/100 WBC.
The blood film from this patient is shown in Plate 3.

Reticulocyte count
8.9%

Hb electrophoresis
HbA 13%
HbA$_2$ 4%
HbF 83%

Questions

Q3.1 What is the most likely diagnosis in this case?

Q3.2 Why is the automated WBC shown incorrect?

Q3.3 How might this be suspected from the appearance of the cell volume histograms?

Q3.4 Calculate the corrected WBC.

Q3.5 What is a pseudogene?

Mark the following True or False.

Q3.6 A. This child is not synthesising β globin.
B. The α globin gene is on chromosome 11.
C. γ globin contains 146 amino acid residues.
D. Most β thalassaemias result from gene deletions.
E. Normal cord blood contains 60-80% haemoglobin F.
F. All globin genes have three introns.

Q3.7 Fill in the names of the missing genes on chromosome 11

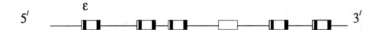

Case 4

Clinical Details

A 30-year-old woman was referred to the gynaecology clinic for investigation of severe menorrhagia.

Clinical examination revealed nothing of significance. On questioning, the woman admitted to bruising excessively on minimal trauma and to have suffered from recurrent epistaxis as a child.

Blood samples were obtained for investigation of a possible bleeding tendency. The results are shown below.

Laboratory Results

Coagulation screen

	Patient	Control
Bleeding time (min)	16	7.5
Prothrombin time (s)	13	13
Thrombin time (s)	11	12
APTT (s)	58	38
Clot solubility	normal	normal

Factor assays

	Patient	Control
IX (IU/dl)	100	103
VIII$_c$ (IU/dl)	12	118
vWF (IU/dl)	20	110
ricof (IU/dl)	18	126

vWF multimeric analysis

All multimers present in reduced amounts.

Platelet aggregation studies

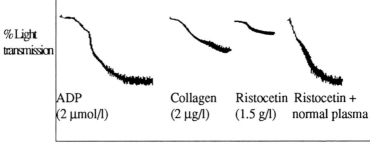

%Light transmission

| ADP | Collagen | Ristocetin | Ristocetin + |
| (2 µmol/l) | (2 µg/l) | (1.5 g/l) | normal plasma |

Time (min)

Questions

Q4.1   What is the most likely diagnosis in this case?

Q4.2   What is the mode of inheritance of this disorder?

Q4.3   The clot solubility test is a semi-quantitative measure of which coagulation factor?

Mark the following True or False.

Q4.4   The following substances are established components in the successful treatment of this disorder:

   A. desmopressin (DDAVP).
   B. heat-treated VIII concentrate.
   C. cryoprecipitate.
   D. anti-fibrinolytic agents.

Q4.5   The following statements relate to von Willebrand's factor (vWF):

   A. it is coded for by a gene on chromosome 16.
   B. it is present in platelet α granules.
   C. it is synthesised by vascular endothelial cells.
   D. its release is stimulated by interleukin-1 (IL-1).
   E. its release is stimulated by vasopressin.
   F. its release is stimulated by prolonged venous occlusion.
   G. platelet adhesion is mediated by low molecular weight multimers of vWF.

Case 5

Clinical Details

A 45-year-old woman presented to her general practitioner complaining of lassitude and a tingling sensation in her fingers and toes. She also admitted to mild weight loss over the previous three months.

Clinical examination revealed moderate pallor and a swollen, inflamed tongue. She appeared to be prematurely grey-haired and had a faint lemon yellow tinge to her complexion. There was no organomegaly or lymphadenopathy.

Blood samples were obtained for analysis. The results are shown below. The full blood count was processed on a Coulter S+IV.

Laboratory Results

WBC	4.6	
LY%	35.7	
MO%	3.3	
GR%	61.0	
LY#	1.6	
MO#	.2	
GR#	2.8	
RBC	2.34	L
HGB	9.3	L
HCT	28.4	L
MCV	121.5	H
MCH	39.7	H
MCHC	32.7	
RDW	19.9	
PLT	144	
PCT	.138	
MPV	9.6	
PDW	16.6	

Cell volume histogram

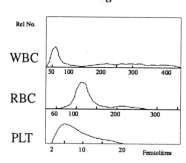

Blood film report

ANI ++
POIK   ++
MACRO ++
Ovalomacrocytosis prominent.
Neutrophils show right shift.
The blood film from this patient is shown in Plate 4.

Haematinic assays

serum vitamin B_{12} 40 ng/l
serum folate   4.9 µg/l
red cell folate   220 µg/l

Auto-immune profile

parietal cell antibodies ++
type I IF antibody ++

Questions

Q5.1 What is the most likely diagnosis in this case?

Q5.2 What is the daily requirement for vitamin B_{12} in a 70 kgadult?

Q5.3 What is the daily requirement for folate in a 70 kg adult?

Q5.4 What is the total body store of vitamin B_{12} in a 70 kg adult?

Q5.5 What is the total body store of folate in a 70 kg adult?

Q5.6 Where is the site of maximal absorption of dietary vitamin B_{12}?

Q5.7 Where is the site of maximal absorption of dietary folate?

Mark the following True or False.

Q5.8   A. Methotrexate is a competitive inhibitor of the enzyme dihydrofolate reductase.
B. Intrinsic factor is a glycoprotein.
C. Transcobalamin I (TCI) migrates with the α globulins on electrophoresis.
D. Transcobalamin II (TCII) is synthesised by granulocytes.
E. Transcobalamin I is 60-70% saturated with vitamin B_{12} in a healthy adult.
F. All cobalamins include a porphyrin ring in their structure.
G. The major cobalamin in human plasma is methylcobalamin.

Case 6

Clinical Details

A 69-year-old man presented to his general practitioner complaining of weight loss, breathlessness and lassitude.

Clinical examination revealed slight pallor and the symptoms of a chest infection. The cervical, axillary and inguinal lymph nodes were enlarged. The swollen glands were firm, discrete and painless. They were distributed symmetrically. The spleen was barely palpable. There was no enlargement of the liver.

Blood samples were obtained for analysis. The results are shown below. The full blood count was processed on a Coulter S+IV.

Laboratory Results

WBC	66.8	H	
LY%	94.1	H	R1
MO%	.7	L	R1
GR%	5.2	L	R1
LY#	62.9	H	R1
MO#	.5		R1
GR#	3.5		R1

RBC	4.88
HGB	15.0
HCT	43.7
MCV	89.6
MCH	30.7
MCHC	34.3
RDW	14.0

PLT	255
PCT	.199
MPV	7.8
PDW	15.5

Cell volume histogram

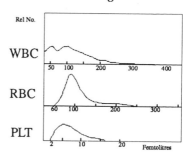

Blood film report

Marked absolute lymphocytosis with numerous disrupted lymphocytes present. No evidence of haemolysis.

The blood film from this patient is shown in Plate 5.

Direct antiglobulin test
Negative

Corrected Hb
13.1 g/dl

Cell marker studies
SIg weak +
M-rosettes ++
CD5 +

Questions

Q6.1 What is the most likely diagnosis in this case?

Q6.2 What is the cause of the disrupted lymphocytes in this disorder?

Q6.3 Cell marker analysis is often performed to identify malignant cell types. For what do these related acronyms stand?

    A. CD antigen.
    B. FITC conjugate.
    C. TRITC conjugate.
    D. APAAP.

Q6.4 Below is a diagram of an immunoglobulin molecule. Match the listed sites to the numbers shown.

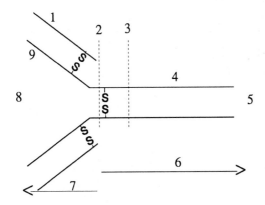

    A. C terminal end.
    B. N terminal end.
    C. Fab fragment.
    D. Fc fragment.
    E. heavy chain.
    F. light chain.
    G. variable region.
    H. site of papain digestion.
    I. site of pepsin digestion.

Case 7

Clinical Details

A 14-year-old boy presented to his general practitioner with a 10-day history of general malaise, lassitude and a persistent sore throat.

Clinical examination revealed symmetrical enlargement of cervical, axillary and inguinal lymph nodes, mild splenomegaly and a pyrexia of 37.8°C.

Blood samples were obtained for investigation. The results are shown below. The full blood count was processed on a Technicon H*1.

Laboratory Results

WBC scattergram

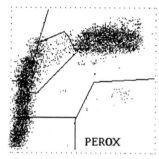

CBC		
6.8	x10⁹/l	WBC
4.56	x10¹²/l	RBC
14.1	g/dl	HGB
42.5	%	HCT
93.2	fl	MCV
30.9	pg	MCH
33.2	g/dl	MCHC
12.3	%	RDW
2.66	g/dl	HDW
246	x10⁹/l	PLT
8.9	fl	MPV

	%	DIFF		x10⁹/l
L	21.1	NEUT	L	1.43
H	59.8	LYMP	H	4.07
	1.9	MONO		.13
	.9	EOS		.06
	.2	BASO		.01
H	16.1	LUC	H	1.10
LI			L	1.78
MPXI				4.0

Blood film report

Absolute lymphocytosis with numerous atypical lymphocytes which are large and have plentiful, deeply basophilic cytoplasm .

Red cells and platelets appear normal.

The blood film from this patient is shown in Plate 6.

Paul-Bunnell screen

Ox red cell stroma	-
Guinea-pig kidney	++

Paul Bunnell titre

Guinea-pig kidney	1/64

Questions

Q7.1   What is the most likely diagnosis in this case?

Q7.2   What is the causative agent of this disorder?

Q7.3   To what group of viruses does this agent belong?

Q7.4   What disease is associated with this virus in central Africa?

Q7.5   What disease is associated with this virus in Southeast China?

Mark the following True or False.

Q7.6   A. B lymphocytes carry membrane receptors for Epstein-Barr virus (EBV).
B. The EBV receptor is CD12.
C. The atypical lymphocytes in this patient are mainly transformed T lymphocytes.
D. Guinea-pig kidney is rich in Forssman antigen.

Q7.7   Complete the following table.

Red cell species	Infectious mononucleosis	Serum sickness
sheep	+	
horse		
ox		
human	-	
guinea-pig		

+ agglutination
- no agglutination

Case 8

Clinical Details

A 15-year-old boy was referred to the haematology clinic for investigation. He had previously presented to his general practitioner complaining of lassitude and pyrexia.

Clinical examination confirmed the findings of the general practitioner viz. pallor and generalised lymphadenopathy. There was no enlargement of the spleen or liver. X-ray examination confirmed the presence of a mediastinal mass.

Bone marrow and blood samples were obtained for investigation. The results are shown below. The full blood count was processed on a Technicon H*1.

Laboratory Results

WBC scattergram

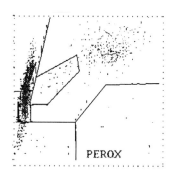

CBC			
H	98.44	x10⁹/l	WBC
L	2.32	x10¹²/l	RBC
L	7.7	g/dl	HGB
L	20.5	%	HCT
	88.4	fl	MCV
	33.2	pg	MCH
	37.7	g/dl	MCHC
H	18.5	%	RDW
H	3.66	g/dl	HDW
L	28	x10⁹/l	PLT
L	5.0	fl	MPV

	%	DIFF		x10⁹/l
L	6.6	NEUT		6.49
H	75.2*	LYMP	H	74.03*
	.3	MONO		.29
	.1	EOS		.10
	1.2	BASO	H	1.18
H	16.6*	LUC	H	16.34
LI				1.33
MPXI				1.9

Blood film report

Marked thrombocytopaenia. Numerous blast cells present, many with atypical morphology.

The blood film from this patient is shown in Plate 7.

Bone marrow report

Hypercellular marrow extensively replaced by type L2 lymphoblasts.

Cytochemistry

Acid phosphatase +++
P.A.S. +/-
Sudan black -

Questions

Q8.1 What is the most likely diagnosis in this case?

Q8.2 What is the nature of the mediastinal mass?

Q8.3 Should this patient be treated as having a good or a poor prognosis?

Q8.4 What substances are stained by the PAS reaction?

Q8.5 What substances are stained by Sudan black?

Q8.6 Which retrovirus is strongly implicated in the aetiology of a variant of this disorder in Japan and the Caribbean?

Q8.7 What property distinguishes retroviruses?

Q8.8 Complete the following table of laboratory results for this disorder:

TdT
Acid phos. + tartrate
SIg
Peroxidase
Chloroacetate esterase
CD2
CD20
CD10
CD7

Mark the following True or False.

Q8.9 The following features are associated with a good prognosis in acute lymphoblastic leukaemia of childhood:

A. white cell count greater than $50 \times 10^9/l$.
B. L1 morphology.
C. hypodiploidy.
D. age 5 years at diagnosis.
E. CD10 positivity.

Case 9

Clinical Details

A 19-year-old woman was referred to the haematology clinic for investigation of a suspected bleeding tendency. She had bled recurrently after a recent dental extraction and claimed to bruise easily.

Obtaining a family history was difficult as her parents had divorced when she was a young child. She thought that one of her mother's sons by her second marriage was a "bleeder". No other conclusive history was obtained.

Blood samples were obtained for investigation and further enquiries were made about her mother and half-brother. The results for all three patients are shown below.

Laboratory Results

Coagulation screen

	Patient	Mother	Half-brother	Control
Bleeding time (min)	6.5	7.5	7.5	5.5
Prothrombin time (s)	13	12	13	13
Thrombin time (s)	11	11	12	12
APTT (s)	72	46	75	40
Clot solubility			All normal	

Both abnormal APTT results corrected by the addition of 1/5th volume of normal plasma.

Factor assays

	Patient	Mother	Half-brother	Control
IX (IU/dl)	115	103	105	110
VIII$_c$ (IU/dl)	8	44	6	100
vWF (IU/dl)	95	110	100	105
ricof (IU/dl)	126	110	110	110

Questions

Q9.1   What is the most likely diagnosis in the half-brother?

Q9.2   What is the pattern of inheritance of this disorder?

Q9.3   What is Lyon's hypothesis?

Q9.4   What is the most likely status of the mother?

Q9.5   What is the most likely diagnosis in the patient?

Q9.6   A family pedigree for this disorder is shown below. Complete
the table for this family.

I1	normal female	II5	
I2	affected male	II6	
II1	affected male	III1	
II2		III2	
II3		III3	
II4	normal male	III4	

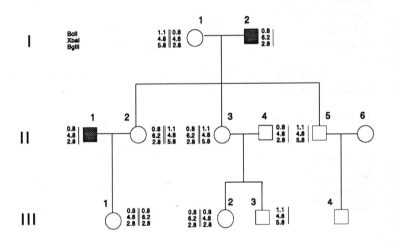

Case 10

Clinical Details

A 65-year-old man presented to the accident and emergency department complaining of severe lower back pain of sudden onset. He had suffered from vague ill health for some months, accompanied by weight loss and anorexia.

Clinical examination revealed moderate pallor and widespread purpura but no enlargement of the liver, spleen or lymph nodes. Radographic examination confirmed vertebral collapse, but also demonstrated diffuse osteoporotic change and well-defined osteolytic lesions in the pelvis and ribs.

Blood and urine samples were obtained for analysis. The results are shown below. The full blood count was processed on a Technicon H*1.

Laboratory Results

WBC scattergram

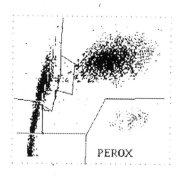

	CBC		
H	15.6	x10⁹/l	WBC
	3.11	x10¹²/l	RBC
L	10.0	g/dl	HGB
	29.1	%	HCT
	93.6	fl	MCV
	32.2	pg	MCH
	34.4	g/dl	MCHC
	13.3	%	RDW
	2.35	g/dl	HDW
L	125	x10⁹/l	PLT
L	6.0	fl	MPV

%	DIFF	x10⁹/l
67.6	NEUT	H 10.54
12.8	LYMP	2.00
1.3	MONO	0.20
.1	EOS	.02
.1	BASO	.02
H 18.1	LUC	2.82

Blood film report
ROULEAUX +++
Blue background stain ++
Plasma cells +
Occ. nucleated RBC present.
The blood film from this patient is shown in Plate 8.

Plasma viscosity
3.85 cP

Protein electrophoresis
Serum
Monoclonal IgAλ band present
Urine
Bence-Jones protein ++

Questions

Q10.1 What is the most likely diagnosis in this case?

Q10.2 What is the cause of the blue background staining on the blood film?

Q10.3 Plasma cells are rich in RNA. What cytochemical method is used to demonstrate this?

Q10.4 What are the primary functions of the rough and smooth endoplasmic reticula?

Q10.5 What is the primary function of the Golgi complex?

Q10.6 Immunoglobulins may be quantitated using Mancini's RID or ELISA. What do these acronyms stand for?

Mark the following True or False.

Q10.7 The following statements relate to IgA:

A. it activates the classical Complement pathway strongly.
B. it crosses the placental barrier.
C. it is abundant in colostrum.
D. it is bound strongly by macrophage Fc receptors.

Q10.8 The following are recognised features of this disorder:

A. the chromosomal abnormality 14q+.
B. raised serum Ca^{2+}.
C. Döhle bodies.
D. renal failure.
E. Russell bodies.
F. "flaming" plasma cells.
G. a peak incidence at 45-50 years.
H. more common in females.
I. platelet dysfunction.

Case 11

Clinical Details

A 36-year-old woman was brought by ambulance to the accident and emergency department. An emergency admission had been requested by her general practitioner who had been called to see the woman by her husband. She had complained earlier that week of general malaise, accompanied by gingival bleeding and bruising.

Clinical examination showed the woman to be extremely anxious, flushed and sweating. She had a pyrexia of 39.4°C and a tachycardia of 115 beats per minute. She had widespread purpura and ecchymoses.

Blood samples were obtained for analysis. The results are shown below. The full blood count was processed on a Coulter S+IV.

Laboratory Results

Cell volume histogram

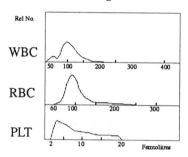

WBC	3.4	
LY%	28.2	R2
MO%	61.5	R2
GR%	10.3	R2
LY#	.9	R2
MO#	2.1	R2
GR#	.4	R2

RBC	2.98	L
HGB	9.0	L
HCT	27.7	L
MCV	92.3	
MCH	30.2	
MCHC	32.5	
RDW	16.6	

PLT	18	L
PCT	.017	
MPV	9.4	
PDW	19.1	

Blood film report

POIK   +
SCHISTO +
Occasional nucleated RBC seen.
Marked thrombocytopenia.
Some promyelocytes show bundles of Auer rods.
The blood film from this patient is shown in Plate 9.

Manual differential count

Neutrophils	2%
Lymphocytes	17%
Monocytes	1%
Myelocytes	19%
Promyelocytes	59%
Blasts	2%

Questions

Q11.1 What is the most likely diagnosis in this case?

Q11.2 The coagulation screen in this patient is grossly abnormal. Why is this?

Q11.3 What are schistocytes?

Q11.4 Why are schistocytes present in this case?

Q11.5 What cytogenetic abnormality is present in virtually all such cases?

Mark the following True or False.

Q11.6 The following statements relate to Auer rods:

A. they are composed of condensed secondary granules.
B. they are stained by Sudan black.
C. they contain myeloperoxidase.
D. they contain alkaline phosphatase.
E. they are commonly present in the blasts of M7 leukaemia.

Q11.7 The following drugs are commonly used in the treatment of leukaemia. Match each with its primary mode of action.

A. methotrexate   1. inhibits topoisomerase II
B. cytosine arabinoside   2. cross-links dsDNA
C. vincristine   3. purine antimetabolite
D. busulphan   4. pyrimidine antimetabolite
E. 6-thioguanine   5. folate antimetabolite
F. etoposide (VP16)   6. disrupts microtubules

135

Case 12

Clinical Details

A 35-year-old man presented to the accident and emergency department complaining of acute epigastric pain, nausea and vomiting. The severity of the pain had increased in waves over the preceding two hours.

Clinical examination revealed abdominal tenderness and muscle spasm in the right upper quadrant, moderate pallor, slight jaundice and a moderately enlarged spleen. Acute cholecystitis was suspected.

Blood samples were obtained for analysis. The results are shown below. The full blood count was processed on a Coulter S+IV.

Laboratory Results

WBC	4.0
LY%	41.3
MO%	2.3
GR%	56.4
LY#	1.7
MO#	.1
GR#	2.3
RBC	2.80
HGB	8.5
HCT	25.2
MCV	90.4
MCH	30.4
MCHC	33.6
RDW	18.5
PLT	185
PCT	.144
MPV	10.0
PDW	16.6

Cell volume histogram

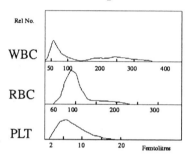

Blood film report
ANI +
SPHERO ++
The blood film from this patient is shown in Plate 10.

Plasma haemoglobin
Patient   6.6 mg/dl
Control   7.4 mg/dl

Osmotic fragility
Patient MCF   5.0 g/l
Control MCF   4.2 g/l

Autohaemolysis test
Corrected by glucose

Questions

Q12.1 What is the most likely diagnosis in this case?

Q12.2 What is the typical mode of inheritance of this disorder?

Q12.3 What is the primary defect in this disorder?

Q12.4 Why is the plasma haemoglobin level normal in this haemolytic state?

Q12.5 Why is the haemolysis corrected by the addition of glucose in the autohaemolysis test?

Q12.6 What pattern of haemolysis is obtained with pyruvate kinase deficient red cells in the autohaemolysis test?

Q12.7 Why has this patient presented with cholecystitis at such a young age?

Mark the following True or False.

Q12.8 The following statements relate to the red cell membrane and its disorders:

A. Aplastic crises are a recognised feature of hereditary spherocytosis.
B. hereditary elliptocytosis is caused by a deficiency of the cytoskeletal protein ankyrin.
C. The cytoskeletal protein band 4.1 acts as a cross-link for spectrin heterodimers.
D. Glycophorin C is associated with the MN blood group antigens.
E. Glucose transport into the red cell is energy-dependent.
F. Glycophorin A is a glycolipid.

Case 13

Clinical Details
A 54-year-old woman presented to her general practitioner complaining of weight loss, anorexia and abdominal discomfort.

Clinical examination revealed pallor and marked splenomegaly.

Blood samples were obtained for analysis. The results are shown below. The full blood count was processed on a Technicon H*1.

Laboratory Results

WBC scattergram

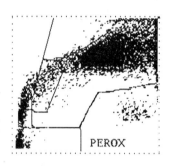

	CBC	
H	100.9* x10⁹/l	WBC
	3.45* x10¹²/l	RBC
	11.6* g/dl	HGB
	34.1* %	HCT
	98.7* fl	MCV
	33.6* pg	MCH
	34.1* g/dl	MCHC
H	21.6 %	RDW
H	3.61 g/dl	HDW
H	547 x10⁹/l	PLT
	8.3 fl	MPV

Values: H 100.9* x10⁹/l WBC; 3.45* x10¹²/l RBC; 11.6* g/dl HGB; 34.1* % HCT; 98.7* fl MCV; 33.6* pg MCH; 34.1* g/dl MCHC; H 21.6 % RDW; H 3.61 g/dl HDW; H 547 x10⁹/l PLT; 8.3 fl MPV

Blood film report
The blood film from this patient is shown in Plate 11.

%	DIFF	x10⁹/l
H 85.2*	NEUT	H 85.97*
8.1*	LYMP	H 8.17*
4.4*	MONO	4.44*
.9*	EOS	.91*
.1*	BASO	.10*
1.3*	LUC	1.31*
LI		L 1.1*
MPXI		6.0*

Manual differential count
Neutrophils	48%
Lymphocytes	6%
Monocytes	3%
Basophils	3%
Metamyelocytes	13%
Myelocytes	20%
Promyelocytes	5%
Blasts	2%

Cytogenetics
t(9q+;22q-) present.

Corrected Hb
10.2 g/dl

NAP score
Patient	9
Control	55

(Normal range 20-100)

Questions

Q13.1 What is the most likely diagnosis in this case?

Q13.2 What is the median survival from diagnosis for this condition?

Q13.3 This disorder typically follows a biphasic or triphasic course. What does this mean?

Q13.4 Why does the manual haemoglobin result (obtained after centrifugation) differ from that obtained by the H*1?

Q13.5 Why is this patient likely to have a markedly raised serum vitamin B_{12} level?

Q13.6 The Philadelphia chromosome results from a reciprocal translocation. What does this mean?

Q13.7 For what purpose is colcemid used in cytogenetic studies?

Q13.8 Individual chromosomes can be identified by the application of G and Q banding. What stains are used in these techniques?

Q13.9 To which group (A-G) of chromosomes does the Philadelphia chromosome belong?

Q13.10 Which two proto-oncogenes are translocated in the Philadelphia chromosome?

Q13.11 Which of these two proto-oncogenes forms a hybrid gene with the BCR gene in the Philadelphia chromosome?

Q13.12 The chromosomal study on this patient is repeated after 6 months when, in addition to the Philadelphia chromosome, trisomy 8 is noted. What is the significance of this finding?

Case 14

Clinical Details

A 20-year-old woman presented to the accident and emergency department complaining of recurrent bleeding from a dental extraction and extensive bruising to the left side of her face. She had suffered from a painful abscess before the extraction of the affected tooth.

Clinical examination revealed nothing of significance. She denied any personal or family history of bleeding or easy bruising.

Blood samples were taken for investigation of a suspected coagulopathy. The results are shown below.

Laboratory Results

Platelet count
   $350 \times 10^9/l$

Coagulation screen

	Patient	Control
Bleeding time (min)	>20	6
Prothrombin time (s)	13	13
Thrombin time (s)	12	11
APTT (s)	35	38
Clot solubility	normal	normal

Platelet function tests

	Patient	Control
Platelet factor 3	normal	normal
Clot retraction	normal	normal
Adhesion	normal	normal

Platelet aggregation studies

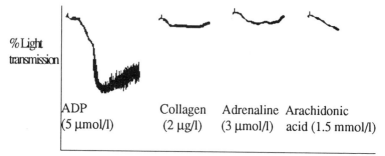

% Light transmission

| ADP (5 μmol/l) | Collagen (2 μg/l) | Adrenaline (3 μmol/l) | Arachidonic acid (1.5 mmol/l) |

Time (min)

Questions

Q14.1 What is the most likely diagnosis in this case? (Hint: remember the patient had suffered from a painful abscess before the tooth was extracted.)

Q14.2 How long is the platelet dysfunction likely to last in this woman?

Q14.3 What platelet enzyme is affected by aspirin?

Q14.4 What is the effect of aspirin on vascular endothelial cell prostaglandin metabolism?

Q14.5 The following statements relate to platelet structure and function. Fill in the blanks.

A. Peripheral blood platelets are _____ in shape and have a mean volume of _____.
B. Platelets survive in the peripheral blood for approximately _____ days.
C. The structure of a normal platelet can conveniently be divided into 4 zones called the peripheral zone, the _____ zone, the _____ zone and the _____ zone.
D. Platelets contain two types of granules. The most numerous are called _____ while the other type are called _____.
E. Platelets contain 2 membranous connecting systems called the _____ and the _____.
F. The dense tubular system is composed of smooth _____ and is thought to be the site of _____ synthesis.

Q14.6 What is the primary defect in the following platelet disorders:

A. Glanzmann's thrombasthenia.
B. Bernard-Soulier syndrome.
C. δ storage pool disease.
D. Grey platelet syndrome.

Case 15

Clinical Details

A general practitioner was called to examine a 3-year-old girl with Down's syndrome by the nurse at her day care centre. The nurse had noted a series of large bruises on the child recently and was concerned about the possibility of "non-accidental injury".

Clinical examination revealed moderate pallor, widespread purpura, bruising and a moderately enlarged spleen. An urgent referral to the haematology clinic at the children's hospital was made.

Blood samples were taken for investigation, and bone marrow aspiration and biopsy performed. The results are shown below. The full blood count on the girl was processed on a Coulter S+IV.

Laboratory Results

WBC	2.0	L
LY%	43.1	R2
MO%	8.7	R2
GR%	48.2	RM
LY#	.9	R2
MO#	.2	R2
GR#	1.0	RM
RBC	3.04	L
HGB	8.0	L
HCT	23.5	L
MCV	77.4	
MCH	26.3	L
MCHC	34.0	
RDW	14.1	
PLT	....	
PCT	....	
MPV	....	
PDW	....	

Cell volume histogram

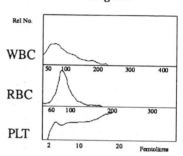

Blood film report
ANI +++
POIK ++
MICRO +
HYPO +
5% blast cells.
The blood film from this patient is shown in Plate 12.

Manual platelet count
42 x 10⁹/l

Bone marrow report
Aspirate - dry tap.
Biopsy - marked fibrotic change.

Cell marker studies
CDw41 +
CD13 +

Questions

Q15.1 What is the most likely diagnosis in this case?

Q15.2 Megakaryoblast maturation is unique among haemopoietic cells. Explain.

Q15.3 What is the name given to this form of mitosis?

Q15.4 What substance is responsible for control of megakaryoblast maturation?

Q15.5 What staining technique is used to visualise bone marrow reticulin?

Mark the following True or False.

Q15.6 The following statements relate to the bone marrow:

   A. it is the main site of erythropoiesis in the foetus at 25 weeks gestation.
   B. A 70 kg adult has about 4 litres of bone marrow.
   C. In chronic myelofibrosis, the marrow fibroblasts are normal.
   D. Foam cells are seen in the bone marrow of patients with Niemann-Pick disease.
   E. A normal adult has irreversibly converted about 50% of their marrow to the yellow, inactive form.

Q15.7 Complete the following table.

Antigen	Distribution	Function
CD2	immature and mature T cells	T cell activation
CD3		
CD8		
CD16		
CD25		
CDw42		

Case 16

Clinical Details

The university medical officer was called as an emergency to the halls of residence to examine a 22-year-old female zoology student. The patient had been unwell for some hours and earlier in the day had complained of a severe headache.

During clinical examination the patient was delirious, sweating profusely and had a pyrexia of 39.8°C. Her liver and spleen were both palpable. She had just returned from a 3-month sabbatical in the Gambia where she had worked in a nature reserve.

Blood samples were obtained for analysis. The results are shown below. The full blood count was processed on a Coulter S+IV.

Laboratory Results

Cell volume histogram

WBC	6.8
LY%	31.4 R1
MO%	. . .
GR%	. . .
LY#	2.1 R1
MO#	. . .
GR#	. . .

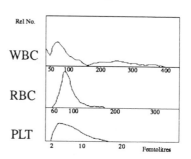

RBC	3.43
HGB	10.2
HCT	30.0
MCV	87.6
MCH	32.8
MCHC	34.0
RDW	16.0

PLT	324
PCT	.224
MPV	6.9
PDW	16.0

Blood film report

Numerous intracellular parasites present in red cells of normal size. Accolé forms and double chromatin dots common.

The blood film from this patient is shown in Plate 13.

Manual differential count

Neutrophils	56%
Lymphocytes	34%
Monocytes	4%
Eosinophils	6%

Questions

Q16.1 What is the most likely diagnosis in this case?

Q16.2 Name the four malarial parasites which commonly infect man.

Q16.3 What is the causative organism of kala azar?

Q16.4 What is the causative organism of Chagas' disease?

Q16.5 What is the likely cause of the high take-off in the WBC histogram?

Q16.6 Match the parasites in the following table to their insect vectors.

A. *Plasmodium vivax*   1. tsetse fly (*Glossina*)
B. *Trypanosoma cruzi*   2. sandfly (*Phlebotomus*)
C. *Leishmania donovani*   3. reduviid bug (*Triatoma*)
D. *Trypanosoma gambiense*   4. mosquito (*Anopheles*)

Q16.7 The following passage relates to the life-cycle of *Plasmodium vivax*. Fill in the blanks.

Malarial infection in man begins when an infected mosquito injects _____ into the bloodstream whilst feeding. These migrate to the liver where they infect hepatocytes and develop into _____, which give rise to the form which enters the bloodstream, the _____. Some of these lie dormant in the liver, when they are known as _____. The most frequently seen intraerythrocytic form is called the ring form or _____, and these develop into _____ which, when mature, release 12-24 _____ which propagate the infection by invading further red cells. Some of these develop into gametocytes and are ingested by a mosquito whilst feeding. The stage of the malarial parasite life-cycle which occurs in man is called _____.

Once ingested by a mosquito the male and female gametocytes fuse to become a zygote. This develops into a motile _____ which bores through the gut wall of the mosquito and forms an _____ from which _____ are released. These are then injected into man while feeding. The stage of the life-cycle which occurs in the mosquito is known as _____.

Case 17

Clinical Details

A 75-year-old man was referred to the haematology clinic by his general practitioner who suspected "something malignant". He complained of shortness of breath on exertion, dizziness, easy bruising. He also suffered from recurrent infections and boils.

Clinical examination confirmed the findings of the general practitioner ie moderate pallor, widespread purpura and an absence of organomegaly or lymphadenopathy.

A bone marrow puncture was performed and blood samples obtained for analysis. The results are shown below. The full blood count was processed on a Coulter S+IV.

Laboratory Results

WBC	4.1	
LY%	49.6	R1
MO%	. . .	
GR%	. . .	
LY#	2.0	R1
MO#	. . .	
GR#	. . .	
RBC	2.88	L
HGB	7.3	L
HCT	20.9	L
MCV	72.8	
MCH	25.3	
MCHC	34.9	
RDW	29.6	H
PLT	. . .	
PCT	. . .	
MPV	. . .	
PDW	. . .	

Cell volume histogram

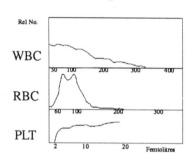

Blood film report

Dimorphic picture with punctate basophilia and occasional nucleated red cells. Numerous hypogranular neutrophils and giant platelets.

Manual differential count

Neutrophils	33%
Lymphocytes	43%
Monocytes	10%
Metamyelocytes	8%
Blasts	6%

Bone marrow report

Hypercellular marrow with severe trilineage dysplasia. Erythroblasts vacuolated and some multinucleate forms present. 15% ringed sideroblasts.

Questions

Q17.1   What is the most likely diagnosis in this case?

Q17.2   What method is used to demonstrate the iron-loaded ringed sideroblasts?

Q17.3   Which organelle is iron-loaded in ringed sideroblasts?

Q17.4   Why does this organelle become iron-loaded in the ringed sideroblasts of sideroblastic anaemia?

Mark the following True or False.

Q17.5   The following statements relate to the sideroblastic anaemias:

   A. Primary acquired sideroblastic anaemia typically presents in infancy.
   B. Ringed sideroblasts are only seen as late normoblasts in primary acquired sideroblastic anaemia.
   C. Chloramphenicol is a known inhibitor of mitochondrial enzymes.
   D. Hereditary sideroblastic anaemia is an autosomal recessive disorder.
   E. Hereditary sideroblastic anaemia is characterised by marked ineffective erythropoiesis.
   F. The presence of ringed sideroblasts is diagnostic of sideroblastic anaemia.

Q17.6   The following features are consistent with a diagnosis of refractory anaemia with excess of blasts (RAEB):

   A. Auer rods present in some of the blast cells.
   B. blast cells absent from the peripheral blood.
   C. at least 25% ringed sideroblasts in the marrow.
   D. a severely hypocellular marrow.
   E. trisomy 8.

Case 18

Clinical Details

A 76-year-old woman presented to her general practitioner complaining of lassitude, a sore throat and severe mouth ulcers.

Clinical examination revealed moderate pallor, a palpable spleen, mild pyrexia and enlargement of the cervical lymph nodes. Her mouth was severely ulcerated and she had hypertrophic, bleeding gums. Antibiotic therapy was instituted and an urgent referral to the haematology clinic made.

Blood and bone marrow samples were taken for investigation. The results are shown below. The full blood count was processed on a Technicon H*1.

Laboratory Results

	CBC		
H	76.6	x10⁹/l	WBC
L	3.02	x10¹²/l	RBC
L	9.2	g/dl	HGB
	28.2	%	HCT
	93.3	fl	MCV
	30.4	pg	MCH
	32.6	g/dl	MCHC
	18.1	%	RDW
	2.89	g/dl	HDW
L	53	x10⁹/l	PLT
	6.0	fl	MPV

%	DIFF		x10⁹/l
L 5.4*	NEUT		4.14*
32.4*	LYMP	H	24.82*
H 12.8*	MONO	H	9.80*
.3*	EOS		.23*
.2*	BASO		.15*
H 48.9*	LUC	H	37.46*

WBC scattergram

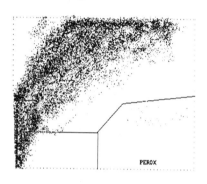

Blood film report

The blood film from this patient is shown in Plate 14.

Bone marrow report

Hypercellular marrow. 70% blasts, promyelocytes and pro-monocytes. Some blasts contain Auer rods. Erythro- and thrombo-poiesis depressed but normal in appearance.

Cytochemistry

Peroxidase	++
Chloroacetate esterase	+
Butyrate esterase	+

Questions

Q18.1 What is the most likely diagnosis in this case?

Q18.2 What is the FAB classification for this disorder?

Mark the following True or False.

Q18.3 The following statements relate to cytochemical staining methods:

A. Non-specific esterases include isoenzymes 3, 4, 5 and 6.
B. α–naphthyl butyrate esterase staining is virtually specific for granulocytes.
C. Fast Garnet GBC is a diazonium salt.
D. Periodic acid oxidises 1,2 glycol groups to dialdehydes.
E. Schiff's reagent consists of basic leuco-fuchsin.
F. Sodium α-naphthyl phosphate is an azo dye.

Q18.4 The following statements relate to the structure and function of monocytes and macrophages:

A. Monocytes adhere strongly to glass surfaces.
B. Macrophages carry three distinct receptors for the Fc portion of IgG (Fc$_\gamma$R).
C. Macrophages carry specific mannosyl-fucosyl receptors which bind non-encapsulated micro-organisms which carry these sugars on their membranes.
D. Fc$_\gamma$RI has a relatively low affinity for IgG.
E. Fc$_\gamma$RIII is synonymous with CD16.
F. The C3b receptor of monocytes is synonymous with CD35.

Q18.5 Complete the following table for this disorder:

Peroxidase	++
Sudan black	
Acid phosphatase	
Periodic acid-Schiff	
CD13	
CD14	
CD33	
TdT	

Case 19

Clinical Details

A 15-year-old boy presented to his general practitioner complaining of extreme lassitude and gingival bleeding. He admitted to chronic solvent abuse.

Clinical examination revealed extreme pallor, widespread purpura and haemorrhagic bullae on the buccal mucosae. There was no enlargement of the spleen, liver or lymph nodes.

Blood samples were obtained for investigation. The results are shown below. The full blood count was processed on a Technicon H*1.

Laboratory Results

WBC scattergram

	CBC	
L	1.0	$\times 10^9$/l	WBC
L	1.98	$\times 10^{12}$/l	RBC
L	5.4	g/dl	HGB
L	16.5	%	HCT
	83.2	fl	MCV
	27.3	pg	MCH
	32.8	g/dl	MCHC
	13.9	%	RDW
	2.98	g/dl	HDW
L	45	$\times 10^9$/l	PLT
	6.1	fl	MPV

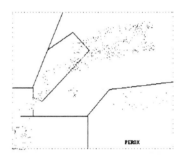

Blood film report

Moderate pancytopenia. No immature white cells seen. Normocytic, normochromic anaemia.

Absolute reticulocyte count

8 × 10⁹/l

8×10^9/l

Ham's test

negative

%	DIFF		$\times 10^9$/l
L	38.7	NEUT	L	.39
	49.8	LYMP	L	.50
	8.6	MONO	L	.09
	.1	EOS		.00
	.1	BASO		.00
	2.8	LUC		1.00
LI			L	1.66
MPXI				.0

Questions

Q19.1 What is the most likely diagnosis in this case?

Q19.2 Which two disorders are characterised by a positive Ham's test?

Q19.3 Bone marrow transplantation is established as an effective treatment for this disorder. Define the following associated terms:

  A. syngeneic donor.
  B. allogeneic donor.
  C. xenogeneic donor.
  D. autologous graft.

Mark the following True or False.

Q19.4 The following are recognised causes of this disorder.

  A. chloramphenicol.
  B. cyanocobalamin.
  C. benzene.
  D. ionising radiation.
  E. Epstein-Barr virus.
  F. non A, non B hepatitis virus.
  G. HTLV-I.

Q19.5 The following statements relate to the HLA system:

  A. The major histocompatibility complex genes reside on chromosome 6.
  B. Class 1 antigens are the products of the HLA-D region.
  C. Class 1 antigens are present on all nucleated cells except spermatozoa and placental trophoblast.
  D. Class 2 antigens are restricted to neutrophils and their precursors.
  E. HLA-B27 is associated with ankylosing spondylitis.

Case 20

Clinical Details

A 33-year-old Greek man presented to his general practitioner requesting screening for him, his wife and son for thalassaemia. His brother had recently been diagnosed as having β thalassaemia.

Clinical examination revealed nothing of significance in either parent. The 12-year-old boy showed significant signs of retarded growth and development, moderate pallor and had a palpable spleen.

Blood samples were obtained from all three patients for analysis. The results are shown below. The full blood count on the boy was processed on a Coulter S+IV.

Laboratory Results

WBC	8.5
LY%	41.1
MO%	3.6
GR%	55.3
LY#	3.5
MO#	.3
GR#	4.7

RBC	6.23	H
HGB	11.0	L
HCT	34.7	
MCV	55.8	L
MCH	17.6	L
MCHC	31.7	
RDW	19.1	

PLT	326
PCT	.241
MPV	7.4
PDW	16.0

Cell volume histogram

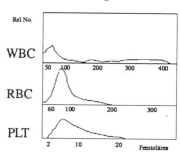

Blood film report
Son

> HYPO +
> MICRO ++
> TAR +
> Occasional nucleated red cell and very occasional irreversibly sickled red cell present.

Haemoglobin electrophoresis

	Father	Mother	Son
HbA (%)	92	60	-
HbA$_2$ (%)	5	-	4
HbF (%)	3	-	8
HbS (%)	-	40	88

Questions

Q20.1 What, precisely, is the most likely diagnosis in the father?

Q20.2 What is the most likely diagnosis in the mother?

Q20.3 What is the most likely diagnosis in the son?

Q20.4 What is a restriction endonuclease?

Q20.5 What is a restriction fragment length polymorphism (RFLP).

Q20.6 What, precisely, is the mutation in haemoglobin S?

Q20.7 Which restriction endonuclease cuts the sickle globin gene at its mutation?

Q20.8 How many exons does a normal β globin gene have?

Q20.9 How many amino acid residues are there in β globin?

Q20.10 What, precisely, is the mutation in haemoglobin Constant Spring?

Q20.11 How many amino acid residues are there in the abnormal globin chain of haemoglobin Constant Spring?

Q20.12 What is the abnormality in haemoglobin Lepore?

Case 21

Clinical Details

A 23-year-old Indian woman presented to her general practitioner complaining of shortness of breath and palpitations. She was 4 months pregnant.

Clinical examination revealed moderate pallor and a smooth, inflamed tongue. Nothing else of significance was noted. During the examination, the patient expressed anxiety about the possibility of thalassaemia in her family.

Blood samples were obtained for analysis. The results are shown below. The full blood count was processed on a Coulter S+IV.

Laboratory Results

WBC	5.80
LY%	33.6
MO%	6.1
GR%	58.4
LY#	2.0
MO#	.4
GR#	3.4

RBC	3.45
HGB	7.4
HCT	24.3
MCV	70.3
MCH	21.4
MCHC	30.5
RDW	17.0

PLT	430
PCT	.370
MPV	8.5
PDW	16.0

Cell volume histogram

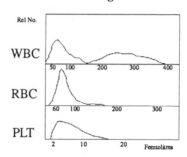

Blood film report
    ANI ++
    POIK   +
    MICRO   +
    HYPO   +
The blood film from this patient is shown in Plate 15.

Iron status
    serum ferritin   6 µg/l
    TIBC   100 µmol/l
    % saturation   9%

Haemoglobin electrophoresis
    HbA 97%
    HbA$_2$ 2.4%
    HbF 0.6%

Questions

Q21.1 What is the most likely diagnosis in this case?

Q21.2 What total quantity of iron is stored by a healthy 70 kg adult male?

Q21.3 What is the site of maximal absorption of dietary iron?

Q21.4 Why would a repeat haemoglobin A_2 and F estimation after suitable therapy be a wise precaution?

Q21.5 What is the discriminant function?

Q21.6 Why is the discriminant function not useful in this case?

Q21.7 Serum ferritin can be assayed using RIA, ELISA and IRMA techniques. What do these acronyms stand for?

Q21.8 Complete the following table:

	Daily loss (mg)	Growth requirement (mg)
infant (6 months)	0.5	0.5
child (8 years)		
adult male		
adult female (25 years)		
adult female (60 years)		

Q21.9 Complete the following table for a healthy 70 kg male:

	% of total iron
haemoglobin	
myoglobin	
haem enzymes	
plasma iron	
body stores	

Case 22

Clinical Details

A 62-year-old man presented to his general practitioner complaining of marked weight loss, sweats and fever.

Clinical examination revealed a markedly enlarged spleen but no lymphadenopathy.

Blood samples were obtained for analysis. The results are shown below. The full blood count was processed on a Technicon H*1.

Laboratory Results

WBC scattergram

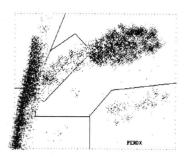

CBC		
H	86.31* x10⁹/l	WBC

	CBC	
H	86.31*	x10⁹/l	WBC
	3.09	x10¹²/l	RBC
	10.6	g/dl	HGB
	28.8	%	HCT
	93.1	fl	MCV
	34.3	pg	MCH
	36.8	g/dl	MCHC
H	19.5	%	RDW
	2.66	g/dl	HDW
L	144	x10⁹/l	PLT
L	6.6	fl	MPV

%		DIFF	x10⁹/l	
L	6.3	NEUT		5.43*
H	65.4 *	LYMP	H	56.45*
	2.6	MONO	H	2.24*
	.1	EOS		.08*
	.3	BASO		.26*
	25.3	LUC		21.84*
LI			L	1.33
MPXI				1.9

Blood film report

ANI ++

MAC +

Mainly normocytic, normochromic. Marked lymphocytosis. Lymphoid cells have plentiful cytoplasm, clumped chromatin and prominent nucleoli.

The blood film from this patient is shown in Plate 16.

Cytogenetics

14q+ present

Cell marker studies

CD22: ++

CD10: -

SIg: ++

Questions

Q22.1 What is the most likely diagnosis in this case?

Q22.2 What is the function of the nucleolus?

Q22.3 What cytochemical method can be used to visualise nucleoli?

Q22.4 Match the disorders to their associated chromosomal abnormality.

A. Burkitt's lymphoma	1. t(15:17)
B. Chronic myeloid leukaemia (CML)	2. t(14;18)
C. M3 (Acute promyelocytic leukaemia)	3. t(8;14)
D. Follicular lymphoma	4. t(9;22)
E. M5a (Acute monoblastic leukaemia)	5. inv(16)
F. M4 (Acute myelomonoblastic leukaemia)	6. del/t(11)(q23)

Mark the following True or False.

Q22.5 The following features are typical of this disorder:

A. raised serum levels of immunoglobulins
B. marked lymphadenopathy
C. raised serum uric acid
D. median age at diagnosis 45 years
E. ribosome lamellar complex on electron microscopy
F. mediastinal mass
G. E-rosette formation
H. CD38 positivity
I. splenomegaly
J. extra-medullary haemopoiesis

Q22.6 The following features are typical of the T cell variant of this disorder:

A. generalised lymphadenopathy.
B. CD2 positivity.
C. CD7 positivity.
D. TdT negativity.

Case 23

Clinical Details

A 17-year-old woman presented to the accident and emergency department complaining of a painful, swollen left leg. This was confirmed by venography to be caused by an ileo-femoral vein thrombosis.

Family history revealed a maternal aunt who had suffered a DVT after a hysterectomy at the age of 46 and that the maternal grandmother had died from a pulmonary embolism at the age of 63. The patient had no history of serious disease which could predispose to thrombosis but had recently been prescribed the contraceptive pill.

Blood was taken for investigation of a possible hereditary prothrombotic state before institution of thrombolytic therapy with streptokinase and heparin. The results are shown below:

Laboratory Results

Coagulation screen

	Patient	Control
Prothrombin time (s)	13	13
Thrombin time (s)	13	12
APTT (s)	35	38
Fibrinogen (g/l)	5.1	2.2

Euglobulin clot lysis time

	Patient	Control
Pre-occlusion (min)	160	140
Post-occlusion (min)	90	80

Protein C assay

	Patient	Control
Amidolytic (u/ml)	1.15	1.20
Immunological (u/ml)	1.10	1.15

Antithrombin III assay

	Patient	Control
Amidolytic (u/ml)	0.60	1.20
Immunological (u/ml)	0.90	1.20

Protein S assay

	Patient	Control
Immunological Free (u/ml)	1.30	1.25

Questions

Q23.1   What is the most likely diagnosis in this case?

Q23.2   Why is there a discrepancy between the amidolytic and immunological assays of antithrombin III?

Q23.3   What is the significance of the woman taking the oral contraceptive pill?

Q23.4   The following passage relates to the structure and function of antithrombin III. Fill in the blanks.

Antithrombin III is a _____ chain glycoprotein which is synthesised in the _____. It has a molecular weight of about _____ daltons. It acts as an inhibitor of coagulation by forming a stable complex with _____ protease coagulation factors, thereby blocking the active site. The complex forms in the ratio of 1 molecule of antithrombin III to _____ molecules of coagulation factor. The rate of formation of these complexes is markedly increased in the presence of the anticoagulant _____.

Mark the following True or False.

Q23.5   The following statements relate to the structure and function of heparin and heparin-like substances:

A. It is most effective as an anticoagulant when administered orally.
B. It is prepared commercially from bovine lung.
C. It is inhibited by platelet factor 3.
D. Low molecular weight heparin has greater antithrombin activity than anti-Xa activity.
E. The plasma half-life of high molecular weight heparin is about 60 minutes.
F. It binds to glutamyl residues in antithrombin III, thus potentiating its antithrombotic activity.

Case 24

Clinical Details

A 24-year-old Thai woman was brought to the maternity hospital as an emergency by ambulance. She was severely toxaemic and in premature labour at 31 weeks gestation. This was her first pregnancy, but she had had no ante-natal care. After a difficult delivery, her baby was still-born.

Clinical examination of the foetus revealed extreme pallor, gross oedema and massive hepatosplenomegaly. The placenta was also grossly enlarged and hydropic.

Blood samples were obtained from both the mother and foetus for investigation. The results are shown below. The full blood count on the foetus was processed on a Coulter S+IV.

Laboratory Results

WBC	+++	H
LY%	. . .	
MO%	. . .	
GR%	. . .	
LY#	. . .	
MO#	. . .	
GR#	. . .	
RBC	2.87	
HGB	5.6	L
HCT	43.1	
MCV	150.1	H
MCH	19.5	L
MCHC	13.0	L
RDW	32.6	H
PLT	. . .	
PCT	. . .	
MPV	. . .	
PDW	. . .	

Blood film report
Mother
    MICRO ++
    HYPO +
    Occasional HbH containing red cell present

Foetus
    ANI +++
    HYPO   +++
    POIK   +++
    nucleated RBC +++

Haemoglobin electrophoresis
Mother

HbA	97.5%
HbA$_2$	2.1%
HbF	0.4%

Foetus

Hb Barts	80%
Hb Portland	17%
HbH	3%

α:β synthesis ratio
Mother
    0.7
Foetus
    no α globin detected

Questions

Q24.1 What is the most likely diagnosis in the mother?

Q24.2 What is the most likely diagnosis in the foetus?

Q24.3 Why is haemoglobin Barts useless as a respiratory pigment?

Q24.4 What has caused the vote-out of the WBC on the foetus?

Q24.5 Complete the following table:

	Genotype
Normal	αα/αα
α thalassaemia-1 trait	
α thalassaemia-2 trait	
HbH disease	
Hb Barts hydrops foetalis	

Mark the following True or False.

Q24.6 A. The coding sequences of genes are called introns.
B. Most α thalassaemias are the result of point mutations within the α gene complex.
C. An acquired form of HbH exists which is associated with myeloproliferative disorders.
D. Most non-deletion forms of α thalassaemia affect the α2 gene.

Q24.7 Fill in the names of the missing genes on chromosome 16.

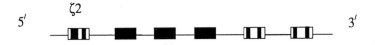

Case 25

Clinical Details

A 6-year-old girl was brought to the accident and emergency department by ambulance. She had complained earlier in the day of a severe headache and feeling generally unwell. The symptoms had steadily worsened and she had suffered a convulsion before the ambulance was called.

On admission, the child was extremely irritable and complained vigorously about the brightness of the lighting. Clinical examination revealed marked pyrexia, neck stiffness and a widespread purpuric rash. She was bleeding from the gums.

Blood and cerebrospinal fluid samples were taken for investigation. The results are shown below.

Laboratory Results

Manual Platelet count
$53 \times 10^9/l$

Coagulation screen

	Patient	Control
Prothrombin time (s)	29	13
Thrombin time (s)	21	11
APTT (s)	64	38
Fibrinogen (g/l)	0.1	2.1
XDP (ng/ml)	1200	100

Blood film report
ANI	++
POIK	+
SCHISTO	++

Neutrophil leucocytosis. Moderate thrombocytopenia.

CSF report
Cell count	6.0×10^6 neutrophils/l
Cocci present	
Gram stain	negative
Total protein	3.0 g/l (Normal range 0.15-0.45 g/l)
CSF glucose	1.3 mmol/l
Blood glucose	4.0 mmol/l

Blood/CSF glucose difference 2.7 mmol/l
(Normal range < 1.5 mmol/l)

Questions

Q25.1 What is the cause of the haemostatic abnormality in this case?

Q25.2 What is the most likely diagnosis in this case?

Q25.3 The following passage relates to the structure and function of fibrinogen. Fill in the blanks.

Fibrinogen is a _____ glycoprotein with a molecular weight of _____ daltons. It is composed of 3 pairs of non-identical chains which are designated _____, _____ and _____. These chains are linked near to the _____ end of the molecule by _____ bonds.

During the conversion of fibrinogen to fibrin, thrombin cleaves two arginine-_____ bonds which results in the release of fibrinopeptides _____ and _____ from the _____ and _____ chains respectively. The resultant molecules of fibrin monomer spontaneously associate. The fibrin clot thus formed is stabilised by the formation of _____ under the influence of factor _____. These form between γ _____ and ε _____ residues, particularly near the _____ end of the _____ chains.

Mark the following True or False.

Q25.4 A. Soluble fibrin monomer complexes can be demonstrated by the addition of protamine sulphate.
B. The XDP test is most sensitive to the presence of fragment E.
C. Fibrinopeptide release is abnormal in fibrinogen Bethesda I.
D. Fibrinogen Oslo is characterised by a shortened thrombin clotting time.
E. The venom of the Malayan pit viper (*Agkistrodon rhodostoma*) cleaves fibrinopeptide A but not fibrinopeptide B from fibrinogen.

Diagnoses for Case Studies

Case 1 This man is suffering from hairy cell leukaemia.

Case 2 The baby is suffering from haemolytic disease of the newborn (HDN) due to ABO incompatibility.

Case 3 This child is suffering from homozygous β^+ thalassaemia.

Case 4 This woman is suffering from type I von Willebrand's disease.

Case 5 This woman is suffering from pernicious anaemia (PA).

Case 6 This man is suffering from chronic lymphocytic leukaemia (CLL).

Case 7 This boy is suffering from infectious mononucleosis.

Case 8 This boy is suffering from acute T-lymphoblastic leukaemia (ATLL).

Case 9 The half-brother suffers from haemophilia A.

Case 10 This man is suffering from IgA myeloma.

Case 11 This woman is suffering from acute promyelocytic leukaemia (APML, M3).

Case 12 This man is suffering from hereditary spherocytosis (HS).

Case 13 This woman is suffering from chronic myeloid leukaemia (CML).

Case 14 This woman is suffering from aspirin-induced platelet dysfunction.

Case 15 This girl is suffering from acute megakaryoblastic leukaemia (M7).

Case 16 This woman is suffering from *P. falciparum* malaria.

Case 17 This man is suffering from refractory anaemia with excess of blasts which, because of the presence of blasts in the peripheral blood is in transformation (RAEB-t).

Case 18 This woman is suffering from acute myelomonoblastic leukaemia.

Case 19 This boy is suffering from aplastic anaemia secondary to solvent abuse.

Case 20 The father is suffering from heterozygous β° thalassaemia, while the mother has sickle cell trait.

Case 21 This woman is iron deficient. A diagnosis of heterozygous β thalassaemia cannot be excluded, however.

Case 22 This man is suffering from B prolymphocytic leukaemia (B-PLL).

Case 23 This woman has antithrombin III deficiency.

Case 24 The mother is suffering from heterozygous α° thalassaemia.

Case 25 This girl has decompensated disseminated intravascular coagulation (DIC).

Answers to Case Studies

Case 1

A1.1 This man is suffering from hairy cell leukaemia.

A1.2 Tartrate-resistant acid phosphatase activity signifies the presence of isoenzyme 5. Although not restricted to hairy cell leukaemia this result is strongly in favour of such a diagnosis.

A1.3 LUC - large, unstained cells.

A1.4 The hairy cells appear in the LUC position of the WBC scattergram.

A1.5
Male : female ratio	4:1
TRAP	+++
SIg	++
E-rosettes	-
Periodic Acid Schiff	-
Butyrate esterase	+
β-glucuronidase	-
CD5	-
CD10	-
CD22	++
CD25	++

A1.6
A. **False.**
B. **False.** Desferrioxamine is a chelating agent.
C. **True.**
D. **False.**
E. **True.**
F. **False.**
G. **True.**

Suggested Reading

Hall and Malia, Chapter 13, The proliferative disorders.
Hoffbrand and Lewis, Chapter 15, Chronic lymphoid leukaemias.

Case 2

A2.1 The baby is suffering from haemolytic disease of the newborn (HDN) due to ABO incompatibility.

A2.2 ABO incompatibility is only rarely severe enough to require exchange transfusion. It is most likely that he will make a complete recovery with no clinical intervention.

A2.3 The risk of HDN due to ABO incompatibility does not increase with increasing parity. The risk in subsequent pregnancies, therefore, is the same as for the general population.

A2.4

	Genotype	Frequency in UK population (%)
R_1r	CDe/cde	31
R_1R_1	CDe/CDe	16
rr	cde/cde	15
R_1R_2	CDe/cdE	13
R_2r	cdE/cde	13
R_2R_2	cdE/cdE	3

A2.5 The mother is most likely to have the genotype rr (cde/cde) and her son is most likely to have the genotype R_1r (CDe/cde).

A2.6

Lectin	Blood group specificity
Dolichos biflorus	anti-A_1
Ulex europaeus	anti-H
Vicia graminea	anti-N
Helix pomatia	anti-A
Fomes fomentarius	anti-B

Suggested Reading

Hoffbrand and Lewis, Chapter 9, Antigens in human blood.
Hoffbrand and Lewis, Chapter 10, Clinical blood transfusion.

Case 3

A3.1 This child is suffering from homozygous β^+ thalassaemia.

A3.2 Nucleated red cells are counted as white cells by this system.

A3.3 The WBC histogram has a high take-off and a prominent population of cells smaller than lymphocytes, resulting in an R1 flag.

A3.4 Corrected WBC = $(100/485) \times 58.8 = 12.1 \times 10^9/l$.

A3.5 Pseudogenes are inactive genes which have a high degree of homology with their functional counterparts but contain mutation(s) which prevent their expression.

A3.6
    A. **False.** He is synthesising HbA.
    B. **False.** The α globin gene cluster is on the short arm of chromosome 16.
    C. **True.**
    D. **False.** Most β thalassaemias are the result of point mutations.
    E. **True.**
    F. **False.** Human globin genes have three exons and two introns.

A3.7

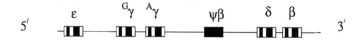

Suggested Reading
Hoffbrand and Lewis, Chapter 5, The haemoglobinopathies.
Hall and Malia, Chapter 9, Microcytic anaemias.

Case 4

A4.1 This woman is suffering from type I von Willebrand's disease.

A4.2 von Willebrand's disease typically is inherited as an autosomal dominant disorder.

A4.3 The clot solubility test is a semi-quantitative measure of the fibrin stabilising activity of factor XIII.

A4.4
A. **True.**
B. **False.** VIII concentrate contains little vWF.
C. **True.** Cryoprecipitate is rich in vWF but is little used nowadays because of the risk of infection.
D. **True.** Anti-fibrinolytic agents are useful in the treatment of menorrhagia..

A4.5
A. **False.** vWF is coded for by a gene on chromosome 12.
B. **True.**
C. **True.** It is also synthesised by megakaryocytes.
D. **True.**
E. **True.**
F. **True.**
G. **False.** Platelet adhesion is mediated by high molecular weight multimers of vWF.

Suggested Reading
Hoffbrand and Lewis, Chapter 21, Normal haemostasis.
Hoffbrand and Lewis, Chapter 23, Inherited bleeding disorders.
Hall and Malia, Chapter 16, Haemorrhagic disorders.

Case 5

A5.1 This woman is suffering from pernicious anaemia (PA).

A5.2 The daily requirement for vitamin B_{12} in a 70 kg adult is 1-3 μg.

A5.3 The daily requirement for folate in a 70 kg adult is about 100 μg.

A5.4 The total body store of vitamin B_{12} in a 70 kg adult is about 3 mg.

A5.5 The total body store of folate in a 70 kg adult is about 10 mg.

A5.6 Dietary vitamin B_{12} is absorbed maximally from the ileum.

A5.7 Dietary folate is absorbed maximally from the upper small intestine.

A5.8 A. **True.**
B. **True.**
C. **True.**
D. **False.**   TCII is synthesised by the liver, ileum and by macrophages.
E. **True.**
F. **False.**   Cobalamins include a corrin ring in their structure.
G. **True.**

Suggested Reading

Hoffbrand and Lewis, Chapter 3, Megaloblastic anaemia.
Hall and Malia, Chapter 2, Physiology of the blood.
Hall and Malia, Chapter 10, Macrocytosis and the megaloblastic anaemias.

Case 6

A6.1 This man is suffering from chronic lymphocytic leukaemia (CLL).

A6.2 The leukaemic cells are excessively fragile and are disrupted during the spreading of the blood film. They are of no prognostic importance.

A6.3
A. CD   Cluster of differentiation antigen.
B. FITC   Fluorescein isothiocyanate conjugate.
C. TRITC   Tetraethyl rhodamine isothiocyanate conjugate.
D. APAAP   Alkaline phosphatase-anti alkaline phosphatase.

A6.4

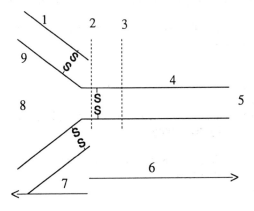

A. 1. light chain.
B. 2. site of papain digestion.
C. 3. site of pepsin digestion.
D. 4. heavy chain.
E. 5. C terminal end.
F. 6. Fc fragment.
G. 7. Fab fragment.
H. 8. N terminal end
I. 9. variable region.

Suggested Reading
> Hoffbrand and Lewis, Chapter 8, Blood group serology.
> Hoffbrand and Lewis, Chapter 15, Chronic lymphoid leukaemias.
> Hall and Malia, Chapter 2, Physiology of the blood.

Case 7

A7.1   This boy is suffering from infectious mononucleosis.

A7.2   IM is caused by the Epstein-Barr virus (EBV).

A7.3   EBV belongs to the family of herpes viruses.

A7.4   EBV is associated with Burkitt's lymphoma in central Africa.

A7.5   EBV is associated with nasopharyngeal carcinoma in Southeast China.

A7.6   A. **True.**
B. **False.**   The EBV receptor is CD21.
C. **True.**   The atypical lymphocytes are activated T cells which are cytotoxic for EBV-infected B cells.
D. **True.**

A7.7

Red cell species	Infectious mononucleosis	Serum sickness
sheep	+	+
horse	+	+
ox	+	+
human	-	-
guinea pig	-	+

+ agglutination
- no agglutination

Suggested Reading

Hall and Malia, Chapter 14, Haematology of infections.
Hoffbrand and Lewis, Chapter 12, Normal lymphocytes and their benign disorders.

Case 8

A8.1 This boy is suffering from acute T-lymphoblastic leukaemia (ATLL).

A8.2 The mediastinal mass is an enlarged thymus gland.

A8.3 T-ALL with a high white cell count and a mediastinal mass at presentation is associated with a poor prognosis

A8.4 The PAS reaction stains substances which contain 1,2-glycol groups eg glycogen.

A8.5 Sudan black stains neutral fats, phospholipids and lipoproteins.

A8.6 HTLV-I.

A8.7 Retroviruses are capable of synthesising DNA from viral RNA within infected cells under the influence of the enzyme reverse transcriptase.

A8.8

TdT	+
Acid phos. + tartrate	-
SIg	-
Peroxidase	-
Chloroacetate esterase	-
CD2	+
CD20	-
CD10	-
CD7	+

A8.9 A. False.
B. True.
C. False.
D. True.
E. True.

Suggested Reading
Hall and Malia, Chapter 13, The proliferative disorders.
Hoffbrand and Lewis, Chapter 14, Acute leukaemia.

Case 9

A9.1   The half-brother suffers from haemophilia A.

A9.2   Haemophilia A is inherited as an X-linked recessive disorder.

A9.3   Lyon's hypothesis states that, early in foetal life, there is a random inactivation of one of the pair of X chromosomes in each cell of a female foetus.

A9.4   Further confirmatory tests are required but it seems highly likely that the mother is a carrier of haemophilia A.

A9.5   The patient is probably an example of extreme Lyonisation in a carrier of haemophilia A.

A9.6
I1	normal female.
I2	affected male.
II1	affected male.
II2	obligate carrier.
II3	obligate carrier.
II4	normal male.
II5	normal male.
II6	normal female.
III1	compound heterozygote female.
III2	carrier female.
III3	normal male.
III4	normal male.

Suggested Reading

Hoffbrand and Lewis, Chapter 23, Inherited bleeding disorders.
Hall and Malia, Chapter 16, Haemorrhagic disorders.

Case 10

A10.1 This is man is suffering from IgA myeloma.

A10.2 The blue background staining is caused by the extremely high level of monoclonal paraprotein in this condition.

A10.3 Methyl green-pyronin (Unna-Pappenheim) staining.

A10.4 The rough endoplasmic reticulum is the site of synthesis of membrane and organelle proteins for the cell and also secretory proteins. The smooth endoplasmic reticulum is the site of synthesis and metabolism of fatty acids and phospholipids.

A10.5 The Golgi complex directs the intracellular transport of membrane and secretory proteins synthesised in the rough endoplasmic reticulum.

A10.6 RID - radial immunodiffusion
ELISA - enzyme-linked immunosorbent assay.

A10.7 A. **False.** IgA activates the alternative Complement pathway.
       B. **False.** Only IgG can cross the placental barrier.
       C. **True.**
       D. **False.**

A10.8 A. **True.** This chromosomal abnormality is common in B cell malignancies.
       B. **True.** This is a reflection of osteolysis.
       C. **False.** Döhle bodies are neutrophil inclusion bodies.
       D. **True.** Acute renal failure is a common cause of death in myeloma.
       E. **True.**
       F. **True.** Flaming plasma cells are seen more frequently in IgA myeloma than other types but are not specific.
       G. **False.** The incidence of myeloma continues to grow with increasing age.
       H. **False.** Myeloma is more common in males.
       I. **True.** Coating of the platelet surface with paraprotein and uraemia both inhibit platelet function.

Suggested Reading
Hoffbrand and Lewis, Chapter 18, Myelomatosis.

Case 11

A11.1 This woman is suffering from acute promyelocytic leukaemia (APML, M3).

A11.2 APML is associated with release of a thromboplastin-like substance from the granules of the abnormal promyelocytes which acts as a trigger for disseminated intravascular coagulation.

A11.3 Schistocytes are fragmented red cells.

A11.4 DIC results in deposition of fibrin in the microvasculature which causes damage to red cells as they pass.

A11.5 The translocation t(15;17) is present in virtually all cases of APML and appears to be a specific finding.

A11.6 A. **False.** Auer rods are condensed primary granules.
  B. **True.**
  C. **True.**
  D. **False.** Alkaline phosphatase is a constituent of secondary granules.
  E. **False.**

A11.7 A. methotrexate   5. folate antimetabolite
  B. cytosine arabinoside   4. pyrimidine antimetabolite
  C. vincristine   6. disrupts microtubules
  D. busulphan   2. cross-links dsDNA
  E. 6-thioguanine   3. purine antimetabolite
  F. etoposide (VP16)   1. inhibits topoisomerase II

Suggested Reading

Hoffbrand and Lewis, Chapter 14, Acute leukaemia.
Hoffbrand and Lewis, Chapter 13, Cytogenetics and leukaemogenesis.
Hall and Malia, Chapter 13, The proliferative disorders.

Case 12

A12.1 This man is suffering from hereditary spherocytosis (HS).

A12.2 HS typically is inherited as an autosomal dominant condition.

A12.3 HS is caused by a deficiency or defect of the cytoskeletal protein spectrin.

A12.4 Haemolysis in HS is primarily extravascular.

A12.5 The defective membrane in HS red cells is highly permeable to sodium ions which must be cleared by increased activity of the ATP-dependent cation pump. The energy required to drive the pump is met by a greatly increased rate of glycolysis within the cell. Haemolysis in the autohaemolysis test results from failure of energy production due to exhaustion of plasma glucose. This failure occurs quickly in HS red cells due to the increased rate of glycolysis. The addition of glucose delays glycolytic failure and so "corrects" the haemolysis.

A12.6 There is no correction of autohaemolysis with the addition of glucose if the glycolytic pathway is impaired.

A12.7 Chronic haemolytic conditions such as HS are accompanied by an increased rate of haem catabolism which leads to increased concentrations of substances such as unconjugated bilirubin in bile. These can precipitate and form pigment stones which may cause cholecystitis.

A12.8 A. **True.** Aplastic crises are often precipitated by infection eg parvo virus infection.
   B. **False.** Hereditary elliptocytosis is caused by a deficiency or defect of spectrin.
   C. **True.**
   D. **False.** Glycophorin A is associated with the MN blood group antigens.
   E. **False.** Glucose transport into the red cell is passive.
   F. **False.** The glycophorins are glycoproteins.

Suggested Reading
Hall and Malia, Chapter 2, Physiology of the blood.
Hall and Malia, Chapter 11, Haemolytic anaemias.
Hoffbrand and Lewis, Chapter 6, Inherited haemolytic anaemias.

Case 13

A13.1 This woman is suffering from chronic myeloid leukaemia (CML).

A13.2 Median survival from diagnosis in CML is 3-4 years.

A13.3 Typically, after 3-4 years in the chronic phase, CML transforms to an acute leukaemia. This transformation may be sudden (biphasic) or may involve a prolonged intermediate or accelerated phase (triphasic).

A13.4 The automated haemoglobin value is obtained in the presence of a large number of white cell nuclei and so is falsely high.

A13.5 Transcobalamin I (TCI) is synthesised by granulocytes. The serum TCI level (and hence vitamin B_{12} level) typically is markedly raised in CML.

A13.6 A reciprocal translocation involves an exchange of genetic material between two or more chromosomes ie some material from chromosome 22 is translocated to chromosome 9 and vice versa.

A13.7 Colcemid is a mitotic spindle poison. It is used to arrest cells in metaphase.

A13.8 G banding results from the use of Giemsa; Q banding results from the use of quinacrine.

A13.9 The Philadelphia chromosome belongs to the G group.

A13.10 ABL is translocated from chromosome 9 to chromosome 22. SIS is translocated in the opposite direction.

A13.11 ABL forms a hybrid gene with BCR on chromosome 22 in the Philadelphia chromosome. The expression of SIS appears to be unaltered.

A13.12 The acquisition of new chromosomal abnormalities often heralds the onset of transformation to the accelerated or acute phase of the disease.

Suggested Reading

Hall and Malia, Chapter 13, The proliferative disorders.
Hoffbrand and Lewis, Chapter 16, Chronic myeloid leukaemia.

Case 14

A14.1   This woman is suffering from aspirin-induced platelet dysfunction.

A14.2   The effect is irreversible and so lasts for the entire life span of the platelets: about 8-10 days.

A14.3   Cyclo-oxygenase is acetylated by aspirin.

A14.4   Acetylation of cyclo-oxygenase blocks synthesis of prostacyclin (PGI_2).

A14.5   A. Peripheral blood platelets are **discoid** in shape and have a mean volume of **6-8 fl.**
   B. Platelets survive in the peripheral blood for approximately **8-10** days.
   C. The structure of a normal platelet can conveniently be divided into 4 zones called the peripheral zone, the **sol-gel** zone, the **organelle** zone and the **membranous** zone.
   D. Platelets contain two types of granules. The most numerous are called α **granules** while the other type are called **dense bodies**.
   E. Platelets contain 2 membranous connecting systems called the **surface-connected canalicular system** and the **dense tubular system.**
   F. The dense tubular system is composed of smooth **endoplasmic reticulum** and is thought to be the site of **prostaglandin** synthesis.

A14.6   A. Glanzmann's thrombasthenia is caused by deficiency of glycoproteins IIb/IIIa.
   B. Bernard-Soulier syndrome is caused by deficiency of glycoprotein Ib.
   C. δ storage pool disease is due to a deficiency of dense bodies.
   D. Grey platelet syndrome is due to a deficiency of α granules.

Suggested Reading
   Hoffbrand and Lewis, Chapter 21, Normal haemostasis.
   Hoffbrand and Lewis, Chapter 22, Platelet disorders.
   Hall and Malia, Chapter 16, Haemorrhagic disorders.

Case 15

A15.1 This girl is suffering from acute megakaryoblastic leukaemia (M7).

A15.2 Megakaryoblasts undergo a unique form of mitosis in which nuclear division but no cellular division occurs. This results in highly polyploid megakaryocytes.

A15.3 This is known as asynchronous endomitotic replication.

A15.4 Megakaryoblast maturation is under the control of the humoral factor thrombopoietin.

A15.5 Bone marrow reticulin is stained by silver impregnation.

A15.6 A. **True.**
B. **True.**
C. **True.** The development of fibrosis is secondary to the development of a neoplastic clone of haemopoietic progenitor cells.
D. **True.** Niemann-Pick disease is one of the sphingolipidoses.
E. **False.** Yellow bone marrow can be converted to active, red marrow if required.

A15.7

Antigen	Distribution	Function
CD2	immature and mature T cells	T cell activation
CD3	mature T cells	T cell antigen receptor
CD8	suppressor T cells	interacts with class I MHC in T cell suppression
CD16	granulocytes and large granular lymphocytes	Fc$_\gamma$RI
CD25	activated T and B cells, monocytes	interleukin-2 receptor
CDw42	platelets	binding of vWF

Suggested Reading

Hall and Malia, Chapter 13, The proliferative disorders.
Hoffbrand and Lewis, Chapter 14, Acute leukaemia.
Hoffbrand and Lewis, Chapter 20, Non-leukaemic myeloproliferative disorders

Case 16

A16.1 This woman is suffering from *P. falciparum* malaria.

A16.2 *P. falciparum, vivax, ovale* and *malariae* all infect man.

A16.3 *Leishmania donovani* is the causative organism of kala azar.

A16.4 *Trypanosoma cruzi* is the causative organism of Chagas' disease.

A16.5 Red cells are lysed in the white cell bath, thus releasing the parasites which register as very small particles in the volume histogram.

A16.6
A. *Plasmodium vivax*   4. mosquito (*Anopheles*)
B. *Trypanosoma cruzi*   3. reduviid bug (*Triatoma*)
C. *Leishmania donovani*   2. sandfly (*Phlebotomus*)
D. *Trypanosoma gambiense*   1. tsetse fly (*Glossina*)

A16.7 Malarial infection in man begins when an infected mosquito injects **sporozoites** into the bloodstream whilst feeding. These migrate to the liver where they infect hepatocytes and develop into **schizonts**, which give rise to the form which enters the bloodstream, the **merozoite**. Some of these lie dormant in the liver, when they are known as **hypnozoites**. The most frequently seen intraerythrocytic form is called the ring form or **trophozoite**, and these develop into **erythrocytic schizonts** which, when mature, release 12-24 **merozoites** which propagate the infection by invading further red cells. Some of these develop into gametocytes and are ingested by a mosquito whilst feeding. The stage of the malarial parasite life-cycle which occurs in man is called **schizogony.**

Once ingested by a mosquito the male and female gametocytes fuse to become a zygote. This develops into a motile **ookinete** which bores through the gut wall of the mosquito and forms an **oocyst** from which **sporozoites** are released. These are then injected into man while feeding. The stage of the life-cycle which occurs in the mosquito is known as **sporogeny.**

Suggested Reading
Hall and Malia, Chapter 14, Haematology of infection.
Roitt, Brostoff and Male, Chapter 17, Immunity to protozoa and worms.

Case 17

A17.1   This man is suffering from refractory anaemia with excess of blasts which, because of the presence of blasts in the peripheral blood is in transformation (RAEB-t).

A17.2   Perl's Prussian blue reaction is used to stain the iron-loaded mitochondria in ringed sideroblasts.

A17.3   See A17.2.

A17.4   The mitochondria are the site of haem synthesis, which is abnormal in sideroblastic anaemia. Mitochondrial iron is under-utilised as a result and so accumulates.

A17.5
A.	**False.**	Primary acquired sideroblastic anaemia typically is a disease of old age.
B.	**False.**	Ringed sideroblasts are seen at all stages of normoblast development in primary acquired sideroblastic anaemia. This is in contrast to the hereditary form.
C.	**True.**	Chloramphenicol is a known cause of secondary sideroblastic anaemia.
D.	**False.**	Hereditary sideroblastic anaemia is inherited as an X-linked disorder.
E.	**False.**	Marked ineffective erythropoiesis is a characteristic of primary acquired sideroblastic anaemia.
F.	**False.**	Ringed sideroblasts may be seen in a wide range of disorders eg leukaemia, pernicious anaemia and acute alcohol poisoning.

A17.6
A.	**False.**	The presence of Auer rods makes the diagnosis of RAEB-t mandatory.
B.	**True.**	Blast cells in the peripheral blood make a diagnosis of RAEB-t mandatory.
C.	**False.**	This is consistent with RAEB-t.
D.	**False.**	The bone marrow typically is normo- or hypercellular in RAEB.
E.	**True.**	

Suggested Reading

Hoffbrand and Lewis, Chapter 9, Microcytic anaemias.
Hall and Malia, Chapter 12, Refractory anaemias.
Hoffbrand and Lewis, Chapter 17, The myelodysplastic syndromes.

Case 18

A18.1 This woman is suffering from acute myelomonoblastic leukaemia.

A18.2 Acute myelomonoblastic leukaemia is designated M4.

A18.3 A. **True.**
B. **False.**   α–naphthyl butyrate esterase staining is present in monocytes.

C. **True.**
D. **True.**
E. **True.**
F. **False.**   Sodium α-naphthyl phosphate is used as a substrate in alkaline phosphatase staining.

A18.4 A. **True.**
B. **True.**
C. **True.**
D. **False.**   Fc$_\gamma$RI has the highest affinity for IgG of the three receptors.

E. **True.**
F. **True.**

A18.5

Peroxidase	++
Sudan black	++
Acid phosphatase	+ (diffuse)
Periodic acid-Schiff	+ (diffuse)
CD13	+
CD14	+
CD33	+
TdT	-

Suggested Reading

Hall and Malia, Chapter 13, The proliferative disorders.
Hoffbrand and Lewis, Chapter 14, Acute leukaemia.
Chanarin, Chapter 9, Morphology and cytochemistry.

Case 19

A19.1 This boy is suffering from aplastic anaemia secondary to solvent abuse.

A19.2 A positive Ham's test is characteristic of paroxysmal nocturnal haemoglobinuria (PNH) and hereditary erythroblast multinuclearity with positive acidified serum test (HEMPAS).

A19.3 A. A syngeneic donor is genetically identical to the recipient eg an identical twin.
B. An allogeneic donor is of the same species but genetically unrelated to the recipient..
C. A xenogeneic donor is from a different species to the recipient.
D. An autologous graft is donated by the recipient.

A19.4 A. **True.**
B. **False.** Cyanocobalamin is a form of vitamin B_{12}.
C. **True.**
D. **True.**
E. **False.** Epstein-Barr virus is the causative agent of infectious mononucleosis.
F. **True.**
G. **False.** HTLV-I is associated with a variant of acute T lymphoblastic leukaemia in Japan and the Caribbean.

A19.5 A. **True.**
B. **False.** Class 1 antigens are the products of the HLA-A, B and C loci.
C. **True.**
D. **False.** Class 2 antigens are found on B cells, activated T cells, macrophages, monocytes, dendritic cells and early haemopoietic precursors.
E. **True.**

Suggested Reading

Hoffbrand and Lewis, Chapter 4, Aplastic anaemia and other types of bone marrow failure.
Hoffbrand and Lewis, Chapter 9, Antigens in human blood.

Case 20

A20.1 The father is suffering from heterozygous $\beta°$ thalassaemia.

A20.2 The mother has sickle cell trait.

A20.3 The son is doubly heterozygous for $\beta°$ thalassaemia and haemoglobin S.

A20.4 Restriction endonucleases are bacterial enzymes which recognise and cleave specific nucleotide sequences in DNA.

A20.5 RFLPs are naturally occurring single base mutations in DNA which either add or remove a recognition sequence for a restriction endonuclease. They are inherited in a simple Mendelian fashion and are useful as markers in linkage analysis of genetic disease.

A20.6 A single base substitution (GAG–>GTG) in codon 6 of the β globin gene results in the formation of haemoglobin S. The abnormality is denoted $\beta6(A3)$ glu–>val.

A20.7 Mst II recognises the sequence CCT NAG G which is present at codon 6 in the β globin gene but absent from the β^s gene.

A20.8 All human globin genes have 3 exons.

A20.9 All non-α globin chains contain 146 amino acid residues.

A20.10 A single base change in the stop codon of the α globin gene (UAA–>CAA) results in translation continuing for a further 31 amino acids.

A20.11 The α globin chain in Hb Constant Spring is 31 amino acids longer than normal ie 172 amino acid residues in total.

A20.12 Hb Lepore is a $\delta\beta$ chain fusion variant. It arises as a result of unequal cross-over between δ and β globin genes. The abnormal globin comprises the N terminal end of δ globin linked to the C terminal end of β globin.

Suggested Reading

Hoffbrand and Lewis, Chapter 5, The haemoglobinopathies.
Hall and Malia, Chapter 11, Haemolytic anaemias.

Case 21

A21.1 This woman is iron deficient. A diagnosis of heterozygous β thalassaemia cannot be excluded, however.

A21.2 Total body iron stores in a healthy 70 kg male are 3-4 g.

A21.3 Iron is absorbed maximally from the duodenum.

A21.4 Iron deficiency can reduce the HbA_2 concentration and cause a diagnosis of heterozygous β thalassaemia to be missed

A21.5 The formula MCV-(5xHb)-RBC-k may be used to help discriminate between iron deficiency and heterozygous β thalassaemia.

A21.6 The discriminant function is unreliable in pregnancy.

A21.7 RIA - radioimmunoassay
ELISA - enzyme-linked immunosorbent assay
IRMA - immunoradiometric assay

A21.8

	Daily loss (mg)	Growth requirement (mg)
infant (6 months)	0.5	0.5
child (8 years)	0.5	0.5
adult male	0.9	0.0
adult female (25 years)	2.3	0.0
adult female (60 years)	0.9	0.0

The daily loss value given for a menstruating female includes an allowance for average menstrual loss.

A21.9

	% of total iron
haemoglobin	65
myoglobin	10
haem enzymes	0.2
plasma iron	0.1
body stores	25

Suggested Reading
Hoffbrand and Lewis, Chapter 2, Iron.

Case 22

A22.1 This man is suffering from B prolymphocytic leukaemia (B-PLL).

A22.2 The nucleolus is the major site of synthesis of ribosomal RNA.

A22.3 Nucleoli contain RNA and so can be stained using the Unna-Pappenheim technique. They can also be demonstrated by their failure to stain with the Feulgen reaction.

A22.4
A. Burkitt's lymphoma	3. t(8;14)
B. Chronic myeloid leukaemia (CML)	4. t(9;22)
C. M3 (Acute promyelocytic leukaemia)	1. t(15:17)
D. Follicular lymphoma	2. (14;18)
E. M5a (Acute monoblastic leukaemia)	6. del/t(11)(q23)
F. M4 (Acute myelomonoblastic leukaemia)	5. inv(16)

A22.5
A. **False.** Immunoglobulin levels typically are low.
B. **False.** Lymphadenopathy typically is absent in B-PLL.
C. **True.**
D. **False.** The median age at diagnosis is 70 years.
E. **False.** This is characteristic of hairy cell leukaemia.
F. **False.** A mediastinal mass is characteristic of T-ALL.
G. **False.** E-rosette formation is a T cell marker.
H. **False.**
I. **True.**
J. **False.**

A22.6
A. **True.**
B. **True.** CD2 is equivalent to E-rosetting.
C. **True.** CD7 positivity is a hallmark of T-PLL.
D. **True.**

Suggested Reading
Hall and Malia, Chapter 13, The proliferative disorders.
Hoffbrand and Lewis, Chapter 15, Chronic lymphoid leukaemias.

Case 23

A23.1 This woman has antithrombin III deficiency.

A23.2 This patient has type II deficiency ie she is synthesising normal amounts of a dysfunctional ATIII.

A23.3 ATIII levels drop significantly in women taking the oral contraceptive pill. This can be sufficient to precipitate thrombosis in women with borderline ATIII levels.

A23.4 Antithrombin III is a **single** chain glycoprotein which is synthesised in the **liver**. It has a molecular weight of about **61,000** daltons. It acts as an inhibitor of coagulation by forming a stable complex with **serine** protease coagulation factors, thereby blocking the active site. The complex forms in the ratio of 1 molecule of antithrombin III to **1** molecule of coagulation factor. The rate of formation of these complexes is markedly increased in the presence of the anticoagulant **heparin.**

A23.5 A. **False.**   Heparin is administered intravenously or subcutaneously.

B. **True.**

C. **False.**   It is inhibited by platelet factor 4.

D. **False.**   Low molecular weight heparin has greater anti-Xa activity than antithrombin activity.

E. **True.**

F. **False.**   It binds to lysyl or tryptophan residues in AT III.

Suggested Reading

Hoffbrand and Lewis, Chapter 21, Normal haemostasis.
Hoffbrand and Lewis, Chapter 25, Thrombosis and antithrombotic therapy.

Case 24

A24.1   The mother is suffering from heterozygous α° thalassaemia.

A24.2   The foetus is suffering from homozygous α° thalassaemia (Hb Barts hydrops foetalis). This condition is incompatible with extra-uterine life.

A24.3   Hb Barts is a tetramer and lacks a Bohr effect.

A24.4   Nucleated red cells are counted as WBC in the S+IV, falsely elevating the WBC to greater than $99.0 \times 10^9/l$.

A24.5

	Genotype
Normal	$\alpha\alpha/\alpha\alpha$
α thalassaemia-1 trait	$\alpha-/\alpha-$ or $\alpha\alpha/$—
α thalassaemia-2 trait	$\alpha-/\alpha\alpha$
HbH disease	$\alpha-/--$
Hb Barts hydrops foetalis	$--/--$

A24.6   A. **False.**   The coding sequences of genes are called exons.
B. **False.**   Most α thalassaemias are the result of gross gene deletions.

C. **True.**
D. **True.**

A24.7

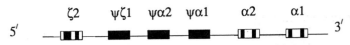

Suggested Reading

Hoffbrand and Lewis, Chapter 5, The haemoglobinopathies.
Hall and Malia, Chapter 9, Microcytic anaemias.
Hoffbrand (1988), Recent advances in haematology 5, Chapter 3, The thalassaemias.

Case 25

A25.1   This girl has decompensated disseminated intravascular coagulation (DIC).

A25.2   She is suffering from *Neisseria meningitidis* (meningococcal) meningitis. This is a common trigger of DIC in children.

A25.3   Fibrinogen is a **dimeric** glycoprotein with a molecular weight of **340, 000** daltons. It is composed of 3 pairs of non-identical chains which are designated Aα, Bβ and γ. These chains are linked near to the **N-terminal** end of the molecule by **disulphide** bonds.

During the conversion of fibrinogen to fibrin, thrombin cleaves two arginine-**glycine** bonds which results in the release of fibrinopeptides **A** and **B** from the Aα and Bβ chains respectively. The resultant molecules of fibrin monomer spontaneously associate. The fibrin clot thus formed is stabilised by the formation of **cross-links** under the influence of factor **XIII**. These form between γ **glutamyl** and ε **lysyl** residues, particularly near the **C terminal** end of the γ chains.

A25.4   A. **True.**
      B. **False.**   The XDP test is specific for D-dimers.
      C. **True.**
      D. **True.**
      E. **True.**

Suggested Reading
      Hoffbrand and Lewis, Chapter 21, Normal haemostasis.
      Hoffbrand and Lewis, Chapter 24, Acquired disorders of haemostasis.
      Hall and Malia, Chapter 2, Physiology of the blood.